Welcome to

THE
EVERYTHING®
PARENT'S GUIDES

As a parent, you're swamped with conflicting advice and parenting techniques that tell you what is best for your child. THE EVERYTHING® PARENT'S GUIDES get right to the point about specific issues. They give you the most recent, up-to-date information on parenting trends, behavior issues, and health concerns—providing you with a detailed resource to help you ease your parenting anxieties.

THE EVERYTHING® PARENT'S GUIDES are an extension of the bestselling Everything® series in the parenting category. These family-friendly books are designed to be a one-stop guide for parents. If you want authoritative information on specific topics not fully covered in other books, THE EVERYTHING® PARENT'S GUIDES are the perfect resource to ensure that you raise a healthy, confident child.

Visit the entire Everything® series at *www.everything.com*

THE
EVERYTHING®
PARENT'S GUIDE TO
Childhood Illnesses

Dear Reader,

As a strong proponent of informative medicine, I like to treat parents as partners. My job is to provide you with the best and most up-to-date facts so you can make an informed decision about your child's health care. This book is a comprehensive compilation of information I routinely use to educate my patients' parents.

Instead of writing another reference book on how to care for a sick child, I decided to focus on addressing the common medical misconceptions. There is already a plethora of pediatric advice books in circulation, and most of them are well written and full of good advice, but there exists a blatant gap in the market for a book addressing myths and fallacies.

As parents, you are constantly bombarded by advice, both solicited and unsolicited. Aunt Mary might object to your letting your children take swimming lessons, and Grandma Mildred might scold you if you leave the air conditioning on at night. Even if you know that some of these things might not be true, you can't really call your doctor whenever such a discussion comes up. If you ever want to find a book that answers such questions with professional medical authority, this book is for you.

Sincerely,

Leslie Young, M.D.

THE
EVERYTHING

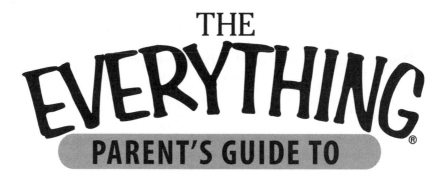

PARENT'S GUIDE TO

CHILDHOOD
ILLNESSES

Expert advice that dispels myths
and helps parents recognize symptoms
and understand treatments

Leslie Young, M.D.
With Technical Review by Vincent Iannelli, M.D.

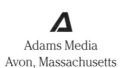

Adams Media
Avon, Massachusetts

For becoming a pediatrician and writing a book for all parents, I am most indebted to my own parents. They have sacrificed much for my brother and me, coming to this country and toiling as immigrants. I can only hope that I have lived up to their expectations and that their hard work has been worthwhile.

• • •

Publisher: Gary M. Krebs
Managing Editor: Laura M. Daly
Associate Copy Chief: Sheila Zwiebel
Acquisitions Editor: Kerry Smith
Development Editor: Jessica LaPointe
Associate Production Editor: Casey Ebert

Director of Manufacturing: Susan Beale
Associate Director of Production: Michelle Roy Kelly
Prepress: Erick DaCosta, Matt LeBlanc
Design and Layout: Heather Barrett, Brewster Brownville, Colleen Cunningham, Jennifer Oliveira

• • •

An Everything® Series Book.
Everything® and everything.com® are registered trademarks of F+W Publications, Inc.

Published by Adams Media, an F+W Publications Company
57 Littlefield Street, Avon, MA 02322 U.S.A.
www.adamsmedia.com

ISBN 10: 1-59869-239-9
ISBN 13: 978-1-59869-239-6

Printed in Canada.

J I H G F E D C B A

Library of Congress Cataloging-in-Publication Data
available from publisher

This publication is designed to provide accurate and authoritative information with regard to the subject matter covered. It is sold with the understanding that the publisher is not engaged in rendering legal, accounting, or other professional advice. If legal advice or other expert assistance is required, the services of a competent professional person should be sought.
—From a *Declaration of Principles* jointly adopted by a Committee of the American Bar Association and a Committee of Publishers and Associations

Many of the designations used by manufacturers and sellers to distinguish their products are claimed as trademarks. Where those designations appear in this book and Adams Media was aware of a trademark claim, the designations have been printed with initial capital letters.

*This book is available at quantity discounts for bulk purchases.
For information, please call 1-800-289-0963.*

All the examples and dialogues used in this book are fictional and have been created by the author to illustrate medical situations.

▶childhood illness n.

1. frequent source of parental anxiety; best conquered with sound knowledge, the guidance of a pediatrician, and—most importantly—the love of a parent.

Acknowledgments

I am indebted to the following people, who supported me through thick and thin during the writing of this book:

My wife, Sherry, who not only tolerated countless hours of late-night typing but also toiled over my manuscript as an editor. My brother Ed, who became my personal legal advisor. My sister-in-law Cindy, who provided me with valuable tips on childhood nutrition. My parents, who inspired all my achievements. My high school teacher, Maggie, who painstakingly proofread my first manuscript. My cousin Mary Ann, who gave me insightful feedback on the earlier drafts of the book. Gina, who believed in my ability as an author. My acquisitions editor, Kerry, who guided me and encouraged me. My development editor, Jessica, who understood my ideas and clarified them. Finally, my friends from the 82saa club, who shared with me their own parenting experiences.

• • •

Contents

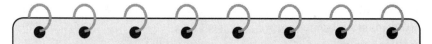

Top Ten Myths about Your Child's Health, Debunked

1. Teething does not cause fever, and high fever cannot directly cause damage to the brain.

2. Natural, 100-percent freshly squeezed orange juice contains more calories than the same volume of nondiet soda.

3. Introducing cereal to your baby's diet early does not make it easier for your baby to sleep through the night.

4. Cracking your knuckles does not cause arthritis.

5. Colic, or excessive crying, has nothing to do with gas or constipation. The gas drops sold to alleviate colic are completely useless.

6. There is no longer any trace of mercury in required childhood vaccines. The link between autism and childhood vaccines has been convincingly discredited.

7. Using hydrogen peroxide to clean a cut can actually impair healing.

8. A green nasal discharge does not mean that your child has a sinus infection.

9. Restricting your child's diet to rice and bananas can prolong your child's diarrhea. Dairy products are perfectly acceptable during a bout of diarrhea.

10. Decongestants and cough suppressants do not alleviate cold symptoms for children less than two years old. Children less than two may suffer serious side effects from these over-the-counter medications.

Introduction

Few occasions provoke more anxiety in parents than when a child is ill, and it is the duty of the pediatrician to calm those parental fears in times of distress. Every day, well-educated and highly intelligent parents unnecessarily bring their children to the emergency room out of fear that a high fever might cause permanent brain damage. Imagine the number of people that might benefit from a book that compiles all these myths and clears up these misconceptions once and for all.

The goal of this book is not to discredit the ancient wisdom of parenthood. The innate instinct of parents often proves uncanny. Indeed, much of the knowledge that has been passed down through the generations has proved to be both practical and life saving. This book is designed to supplement experience and instinct to empower parents with the latest, most accurate medical information. This allows you to make the best decision for your children when they are not feeling well.

While instinct and experience are often valuable, there are also numerous myths associated with children's health. Though the origin of most of these misconceptions is obscure and lacking in supporting evidence, they tend to be tenaciously held by many parents.

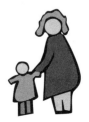

The idea for this book, which covers conditions that affect infants to adolescents, was born from a desire to shed light on these areas of misunderstandings. This book is intended for all parents, as well as for people who plan to become parents one day. It is not just intended for new parents; many of the myths addressed in the book are widely believed, even by experienced parents who have raised many children. In fact, grandparents can also benefit from this book, as they are frequently the source for advice in child rearing.

This book is not intended to serve as a comprehensive reference book concerning the care of your child. Rather, it is meant to complement medical source books such as those. It is written to address subjects that are not often covered by books on pediatric health. A typical parent with children is likely to be too tired to read another comprehensive manual on how to raise children. Most parents are lucky to garner enough energy to make it through the day without collapsing. Raising children is rewarding, but it can be extremely taxing at the same time. This is a book that parents can read for fun while their princes and princesses are taking their afternoon naps. Not only does it provide an interesting read, it also educates parents in a condensed format on how to better care for their loved ones.

Because this book is not written for medical professionals, no prior medical knowledge is required to read and understand the content. In fact, one of the aims of this book is to translate inaccessible information and make it available to every parent.

Lastly, this book was purposely designed to have a light tone and to be easy to read. Dealing with a sick child is stressful enough. While some of the subject matter covered here is serious and heavy-duty stuff, the content is infused where appropriate with humor and levity. This is definitely not a cut-and-dried medical textbook. At all times, the information is relevant to the reader and readily applicable to real-life situations.

CHAPTER 1

How to Find a Good Pediatrician

C hoosing your child's doctor might be one of the most important decisions you'll have to make as a parent. If you find the right pediatrician, you will have a knowledgeable ally by your side through thick and thin. If not, you might find yourself fighting an uphill battle with the health-care system. This chapter will guide you through the tricky business of finding the right doctor.

The Perfect Match

On the surface, all doctors might seem to be equal. After all, they have all gone through the rigors of medical school and survived a grueling residency training process. In addition, their competency is ensured by each state's medical board when they receive certification in their specialties. However, doctors are human, and despite the similarities in their medical training, they retain their individuality. Finding the right doctor does not simply mean getting someone who meets the standard qualification of providing health care; rather, it is about finding someone you can relate to and trust.

A Matter of Style

Doctors have their own traits and idiosyncrasies, and they will inevitably bring these individual characteristics into their practices. The way they interact with patients and parents, follow up on their patients' conditions, and prescribe medications are all influenced by their personalities. While doctors do perform within the bounds of what is acceptable in the medical community, there is still a lot of room for personal judgment. This is why medicine is sometimes considered an art as well as a science.

Similarly, parents come in all varieties too. Their personal predilections also influence their child-rearing styles and parenting techniques. Though there is no right or wrong way of doing most things, differences in opinion can cause some interesting debates. Consequently, the task at hand is to find a physician who understands you and to whom you can relate. Personality does go a long way when it comes to picking out the right doctor. Aside from proper training and technical competence, a good personality match is the foundation of a good parent-doctor relationship.

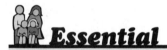 **Essential**

Finding the right doctor is not too different from finding your soul mate. Sometimes the most important factor is that elusive chemistry between two individuals. You might not feel comfortable with a doctor, even though his credentials are impeccable and he is perfectly charming. If you do not feel that sense of chemistry with your doctor, the parent-doctor relationship can be compromised.

What should you look for in terms of personality? In general, there are two major styles of practice when it comes to medicine. In the past, the relationship between the patients and physicians was mostly paternalistic. In other words, doctors acted in a "father knows best" fashion. In this type of relationship, the doctor dictated what needed to be done, and the patient complied without asking a lot of questions. This style of medicine allowed only for one-way communication. It worked fairly well for patients who had great confidence in their doctor's skills, which tended to ensure that they would comply with recommended treatments.

The other style of medical practice can be described as informative. As the paternalistic style slowly goes out of favor with the general public, the informative style is gradually taking hold as the predominant type of patient-physician relationship. In this type of practice, the physician establishes a partnership with the patient and acts as a trusted source of information. The doctor's task in this case is not to dictate what to do but to educate the patient about various treatment options. Ultimately, the doctor empowers his patients and allows them to reach an informed decision about their own health conditions.

From these descriptions alone, most readers can easily pick out the type of practice that is most comfortable for them. Most people would think that the choice between these opposite styles was a no-brainer. In reality, you would be surprised at the number of people who opt for the other choice. There is nothing wrong with either style. As long as it fits your personality, you will feel right at home with the choice you make.

A Matter of Speaking

The way a doctor speaks could be just as important as her style of practice. Some doctors are soft-spoken and gentle, while others are loquacious and confident. Even if they utter the exact same words, they can leave drastically different impressions.

Many parents are inclined toward doctors who are talkative and friendly. They feel at ease chatting with the doctor about home-improvement projects or last night's football game. A rapport can be quickly established, especially if the doctor has interests and hobbies in common with the parents. This feeling of familiarity and comfort serves as a building block for the trust between doctors and parents when it comes to making important medical decisions.

Other doctors are more reserved and conservative, which some parents prefer because they interpret this as a professional demeanor. If the doctor seems too friendly, the parents' confidence in her professionalism could be shaken. Patients who feel more comfortable with the paternalistic approach may prefer this type of doctor.

Finally, for many patients and parents who speak a language other than English, the paramount criterion is to find a doctor who can speak their native tongue. A language barrier can prevent seamless information exchange. Even with the help of a good translator, a lot of details in the description of the illness and treatment instruction can be lost. In addition, a professionally trained translator is not always readily available. In such scenarios a medical visit is often reduced to the bare essentials. This situation definitely does not allow the doctor to do her best work.

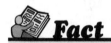 **Fact**

More and more physicians are learning a second language to better communicate with a greater number of their patients and parents. While medical translators are often readily available, getting an important message across through a third person increases the probability that details will be lost in translation. In addition, it is significantly more difficult to establish rapport via a translator.

Cultural Differences
Sometimes it's not enough for the doctor to just speak a patient's language. It's also necessary to understand the context of the ideas and facts being conveyed. Literal understanding of the words may not convey the real meaning behind the

conversation. A doctor who can appreciate the nuances of your culture can be valuable indeed.

Most people are aware of cultural differences when it comes to health and healing. Every culture harbors its unique set of beliefs and practices. Bringing these to a doctor who is foreign to the culture may not only lead to misunderstandings, it can sometimes have unfortunate consequences for the family as well.

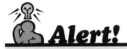

Alert!

While most cultural folk remedies are benign, some practices can harm your child. When in doubt, ask your pediatrician before performing any treatments that are not endorsed by Western medical standards.

Where to Look

After you have decided on the type of doctor you prefer, the next question is how to find her. Resources are plentiful in today's digital world, but using them properly and efficiently can be tricky. This section will explore the possibilities and assist you in finding the doctor of your dreams.

The Internet

The Internet has consolidated a large collection of human knowledge in the past decade. Use it wisely, and you will reap the treasures that are stored in its trove; be careless, and risk being abused and misled. In fact, most physicians use the Internet as an important way of keeping pace with medical advances as well as a comprehensive reference. In addition, many cutting-edge clinical research institutions announce their latest findings on the Internet.

One of the best resources on the Internet is the database each state keeps of medical board physicians. This vastly under-publicized but free information is extremely valuable. Basic information is listed for the physician, including address and telephone number. The best way to find this database in your state is to do an Internet search for the keywords "state medical board" and the name of your state.

Many states also display how long the physician has been in practice and what medical school the physician graduated from. However, the most useful information is whether the physician has been the target of any professional disciplinary action. This includes any lawsuits, probation, license suspension, revocation, or other more minor warnings, either in the past or present. Almost all states have at least a searchable database for the public, and all that is needed to complete a search is the name of the physician.

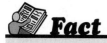 **Fact**

Unfortunately, each state medical board has its own Web site, so there is no centralized location where patients can do a search on physicians throughout the country. You can find the Web site for your state's medical board by using the keywords "state medical board" and the name of your state in your search.

The main problem with this database is that information is not universally available. Each state manages its own database, so the format and the information available vary between states. In some states, the information is privileged, and the consumer has no easy way of obtaining it from the Web site. This may change in the future, however, as more and more states jump onto the bandwagon to empower consumers.

While there is no single Web site that contains physician data for all the fifty states, the American Medical Association Web site (at *www.ama-assn.org*) includes links to the individual sites for all the state medical boards. The format of these sites varies greatly from state to state.

The Friend

If you have children or are planning to have them, chances are that you have friends with children as well. One of the best sources of information regarding pediatricians is word of mouth from your friends and relatives. Knowing the personality of your friends and family, you can gauge whether their doctor will work for you too.

Keep in mind that what works for them may not work for you, even if your personalities are similar. Ask your friends exactly what they like about their doctors. Ask for specific examples, like the doctor's patience when she explains how to use a particular medication or how she invariably calls on the following day to check up on the condition of your children. These little things can paint a clear picture of the doctor and what she is like.

The Referral

Even if your friend or family member can't help you find the doctor you want, her doctor might be able to recommend a colleague who might fit your personality better. Most doctors don't mind referring patients to another doctor, especially if they feel that another physician can provide a better fit for the patient and parents.

The best way to accomplish this is to visit the doctor your friend recommends. You can also simply go to a doctor you pick out from the list of those available under your insurance plan. At the end of the visit, if you still prefer another doctor, you can politely ask the doctor for a physician recommendation. This is done routinely, and the doctor should not be offended by your request.

Age and Sex

Even after you have found your perfect doctor, this does not mean the search is over forever. As your children grow and mature, they might develop preferences of their own. For instance, they might decide they prefer either a male or female physician. It is not as simple as matching up the gender of your child with the doctor of the same gender. You might be surprised to learn, for instance, that your adolescent son would rather have a female than a male physician.

The gender of the physician is most relevant when it comes to certain types of exams. As you can imagine, it might be somewhat awkward for a teenage girl to go to a male doctor for problems relating to her breasts or reproductive organs. Similarly, some boys might be uncomfortable with a female doctor when they are visiting the office for issues concerning their private parts. All these must be taken into consideration.

When to Switch

How do you know when to choose another doctor if your child doesn't come up and tell you directly? It may seem obvious, but the best way is to ask your child. The best time to ask is when your child has reached the age of ten or so. Most children of this age are opinionated enough to want to make certain choices in their lives. You cannot assume your children will raise this issue on their own, as they might not be aware that they have the option of choosing or changing doctors unless you present it to them.

Age of the Doctor

This is a tricky area of discussion. Parents often believe that young doctors lack the clinical experience of older physicians. On the flip side, others worry that older doctors may not keep up with the latest medical advances and changing treatment guidelines. Even though there might be a grain of truth in this concern, either one of these judgments is unfair in most circumstances.

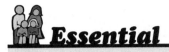

Essential

While the age of the doctor is worth considering, it is arguably one of the least important factors in choosing a physician. If you feel very comfortable with a doctor, it's probably best to stick with her no matter how old or young she may be. A good doctor is hard to find, and a good doctor who works well with you is even harder to find.

For any physician to become an independent practitioner, he must go through years of residency training, during which he practices medicine under the strict supervision of experienced senior physicians. By the time he finishes residency, he has been taking care of patients for many years and making his own medical decisions. The intensity of this training process ensures that no one finishes the program without garnering enough experience to confidently practice medicine independently.

On the other end of the age scale, there is another system that ensures that older physicians do not fall behind in learning up-to-date medical technology. All physicians are required to attend educational seminars regularly, and all major hospitals require their doctors to submit proof that they have attended a certain number of these meetings. In addition, in order to maintain certification in a medical specialty such as pediatrics, the law usually mandates that practitioners take a recertification examination every seven years to keep their license active. Through this vigorous set of checks and balances, the standard of medical care in this country is always upheld.

At the same time, it would be wrong to say that the age of the physician should never be considered as a factor when you're choosing your doctor. Your child may feel more comfortable with either a younger or older physician, based on your past experience. Commonsense considerations also play a part here. For instance, it is probably not a good idea to select a doctor who is scheduled to retire within the next six months.

Consider the Location

Even if you have found the world's greatest doctor, seeing her could still be an unpleasant experience if you have to drive a long distance for each office visit. In addition, a long drive would effectively preclude you from bringing your children to the doctor in case of an emergency. Needless to say, proximity is an essential factor when deciding on your child's doctor.

Proximity to your residence is not the only consideration when it comes to location. Sometimes it may be easier for you to pick up your daughter from day care or school and bring her directly to the doctor. If the doctor's office is located near the school, it may be more convenient for you to select that particular office for routine visits.

The flow of traffic may also be a determining factor. In many urban centers in this country, traffic congestion has become a part of city dwelling. It may make more sense to select an office that is situated in a part of town that lets you drive against the major flow of traffic than to select another office that is closer but less accessible due to bad traffic.

Availability Is Essential

Availability can be a Catch-22. Many of the most popular doctors have established a large patient base, and their schedule is booked four to six months in advance. In this case, even if the doctor you select is the most convenient and compatible around, you'll probably never see him because of his busy schedule. If his schedule doesn't accommodate your needs, the kind of rapport you strike up with each other is irrelevant.

Office Hours

Not only does the doctor have to be available, he has to be available at a time that is convenient to you. It doesn't matter if his schedule means his office is open from nine to five if you have to be at work during those hours. If your only free time is after five, when this particular doctor has already stopped seeing patients, you'll never get to see him. You probably will end up seeing his colleagues most of the time. This defeats the purpose of carefully picking your doctor out of the crowd in the first place.

Call the office to get some ideas of office hours and a given doctor's availability. Not all doctors work regular hours. Some routinely work late once or twice a week, and that could work in your favor.

Your doctor may be great, but if he only works three days a week and takes four month-long vacations a year, you may find yourself stranded most of the time. Ideally, you should find out this information not only from the office staff, but from other patients.

After Hours

For many parents, a pediatrician's availability after hours is a deal breaker when it comes to choosing their child's doctor. In the past, when private practices were the norm, most doctors took calls daily. This meant that patients could count on reaching their doctor in case they had an urgent question, even after the office was closed.

With a changing health-care system and the proliferation of group practices, this easy availability of doctors has become a rarity. Large organizations such as hospitals and clinics usually set up a telephone nurse triage system that parents can use to get most general questions answered at any time of day or night. However, this service does not provide the personalized care of the old system. The person on the other end of the phone does not know the subtle nuances of your child's health condition in the way your own pediatrician does.

Inquire about the on-call system and the availability of the doctor when you are shopping for a practice. This could mean the difference between a delay in treatment or an unnecessary trip to the emergency room.

Even if your pediatrician does not provide after-hours care, she can usually recommend several local urgent-care facilities as alternatives. Some of these neighborhood urgent-care clinics are actually underused because they are not widely publicized.

If you do not have medical insurance, there are still options available for you, although your selection is more limited. There are some government-sponsored clinics that stay open after hours on certain weekdays. These might not be located in your neighborhood, so you may have to drive farther to reach them. Once again, your pediatrician is the most knowledgeable person you can ask for information about any clinics that might be located near your neighborhood.

CHAPTER 2

Baby Issues

After nine long months of pregnancy, your bundle of joy is finally here. It isn't until you get home from the hospital with your tiny newborn that you realize something is missing. Where is the official manual? There is certainly no shortage of advice. Grandmother sternly advises you to bundle the baby up in four layers of wool blankets. Your aunt, on the other hand, tells you to give the baby some water because the weather is so hot. Who do you listen to?

Exposure to the Elements

Newborn babies seem so fragile. They're so tiny, their skin so soft and their cry so desperate. It seems that every little thing has the potential to cause them harm. Your parental instincts tell you to keep your baby safe and protected from everything, even things that seem innocuous. In fact, doctors used to recommend that parents keep their newborn infants at home for three weeks after birth (not something you're likely to hear from you pediatrician these days). The following sections describe what level of vigilance is appropriate and what is going overboard.

Overprotection

Even though it is a good idea to try to keep your newborn from getting sick, it is unnecessary to quarantine her completely. Many traditional beliefs dictate that new parents keep from taking a new baby outside of the house at all. For new parents who are already overwhelmed with the responsibilities of taking care of a new infant, cutting off the outside world completely only adds to stress levels.

Why did people used to think it unwise to take a new baby outside? There are two possible reasons. First, an infant's skin is extremely prone to sun damage. A baby can get a sunburn in less than five minutes under direct sunlight, even in the weakened morning sun. However, there is no reason that you cannot bring the baby outside while protecting him from direct sunlight. You can safely put your newborn in a completely shaded stroller and enjoy a nice walk in the park. A simple activity like this can mean the world to an exhausted new parent.

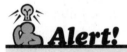

Alert!

Even though a new baby is very sensitive to sunlight, you cannot apply sunscreen to her skin until she is six months old. Until that age, a baby's skin is sensitive to the active ingredient in sunscreen. Exposing a too-young infant to this chemical might make her skin to break out in an allergic rash.

The second reason behind the myth that babies should be kept indoors is fear that the baby might get sick. Unless it's a crowded place in the middle of the flu season, the outside air is not contaminated with germs. Contrary to what most people believe, most infections are not transmitted through the air. The vast majority of infections, including the common cold, are transferred from one person to the next by contact alone, a method of infection known as contact transmission. The best way to keep your baby healthy is simply to wash your hands.

Underprotection

There are some exceptions to the rule of contact transmission. Some serious infections are passed around by airborne particles. The flu is one of the most common infections that can be transmitted this way. Measles and chickenpox are also notorious for their ability to infect their victims without contact. It is still a good idea to avoid sick people when you are carrying your newborn around. If you know someone is sick, don't allow that person to come over and see the baby. Furthermore, it's a good idea to keep the number of people who handle the baby to a minimum. Ideally, no more than two people other than the parents should directly touch the baby. Strictly following this recommendation should drastically reduce the chance that the baby catches a bug in the first month.

Some people raise their babies without worrying too much about infection. Their reasoning is that they do not want their children to be too "delicate." Instead, they want their children to be exposed to germs early on so they will not get sick later. This is another error in thinking. The newborn period is not the best time to build up the immune system in a child.

During the first few months, the immune system of an infant is significantly weaker than that of an adult. Consequently, doctors tend to become very concerned if a baby less than a month old gets a fever. If the baby has a rectal temperature of 100.4°F or more, he will most likely be sent to the hospital for a spinal tap so doctors can rule out an infection of the brain. Fever in children older than a year old is much less dire, and infection control is much less of an issue in these older children.

The Cold Air

A baby cannot get sick from pure exposure to cold air. It is unnecessary to bundle a baby up in many layers. In fact, this might cause the baby to overheat, which could be a serious issue. Instead of excessive bundling, you should dress the baby in the same number of layers that you dress yourself.

Similarly, air-conditioning on its own cannot cause a baby to come down with a cold. On a hot day, it is actually a good idea to keep the baby in a cool, air-conditioned room. The only potential harmful effect of air-conditioning is that it tends to recirculate the indoor air, thus making airborne infections more communicable.

Those Baby Blues

Being one of the most notable body parts, the eyes of the baby capture a lot of attention from new parents. Every little thing with the eyes tends to get noticed immediately. This section covers some of the most common conditions that can affect the eyes of a newborn. Fortunately, most of these conditions are harmless and do not pose any permanent problem for the baby.

Bleeding

As a result of the tremendous pressure exerted on a baby's head during her journey through the birth canal, many babies end up with minor leaks of the small blood vessels in the eyes. This may sound scary and dangerous, but it is entirely harmless. You may notice a bright red spot with irregular edges in the white part of the eye, sometimes directly adjacent to the iris. The red patch is usually small, but it can also be quite large, covering most of the white. This can happen in one eye or both.

The bleeding never affects the baby's vision. It is completely painless, and the redness generally disappears in less than two weeks. Nothing can be done to make the redness go away sooner. Regardless of how it looks, it is never a serious problem. You do not have to do anything to it to make it go away. If you are still concerned, you can specifically ask the pediatrician to check the bleeding during the baby's first exam.

Eye Mucus

In many babies, parents may notice a sticky, yellowish discharge from either one of the eyes or both. This can happen soon after birth or after a few weeks. Usually, the eye that has the discharge is watery, and the eyelid may become slightly swollen as well. The baby does not behave in a way that indicates he feels unwell.

This condition occurs when the small tube that drains tears from the eye is temporarily blocked. Everyone's eyes are equipped with this small drainage system. Eyes constantly produce tears to moisten and lubricate the eyeballs, and this small amount of tears drains into the nose via small tubes that connect the eye and the nasal passage.

Just like the rest of the baby, these small drainage tubes are tiny compared to their counterparts in adults. They often get clogged or blocked. The blockage may come and go over a period of several months. Parents can help unclog these ducts by massaging the area between the bridge of the nose and the eye with a clean towel soaked in warm water. Take care not to apply pressure directly to the eye, as that can damage the delicate eyeball.

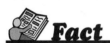 **Fact**

If blockage of the tear ducts persists past the first year of life, the pediatrician usually refers the baby to an eye specialist, who will attempt to open up the duct slightly using precise instruments. This is usually not necessary. For the vast majority of babies, the condition resolves in less than nine months.

Many parents believe this is a sign of eye infection, and, unfortunately, many health-care professionals perpetuate that belief by treating the condition with antibiotics. True infection of the eye does happen in newborn babies, but it is rare compared to this relatively common condition. As long as the eye discharge does not occur simultaneously with redness of the white part of the eye, you can be confident that there is no infection present.

On the other hand, if you notice that the whites of your child's eyes are bloodshot and you also find copious, thick discharge from the eyes, you should contact your doctor immediately. If the mother has a history of certain STDs, her infection may have spread to the baby's eyes during labor and delivery. If these infections go undetected and untreated, the baby may lose her eyesight.

Skin and Rashes

It is ironic that so many people envy the softness of a baby's skin when the skin of a baby is frequently afflicted by all sorts of strange rashes and blisters. This contradiction in people's perception can cause parents to become alarmed when their baby's smooth skin gets blotchy and discolored. It is especially a source of concern when these rashes appear in unusual patterns—these often have no equivalents in adult skin ailments.

Peeling Skin

Most babies are born with relatively smooth skin, but almost immediately that smoothness gives way to significant peeling. The skin around the feet and the abdomen is especially prone to this peeling, but it can happen to skin all over the body. This is particularly common for babies who are born after their due dates; it is rare in premature infants.

Faced with a skin problem like this, the first natural impulse of most parents is to put gobs of moisturizer onto the skin because the peeling skin appears dry. Pediatricians, however, recommend against such practice. Even though the peeling skin is unsightly, the underlying skin is not really dry. It does not need to be moisturized.

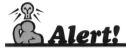

Alert!

It is generally not recommended for parents to use lotions or baby oils until the baby is at least a month old. Using these products too early may cause an allergic reaction because a baby's skin is so sensitive.

Indications of a Serious Condition

There are two common skin conditions in the newborn that are particularly dangerous. You need to seek medical attention immediately if you notice a rash that fits the following descriptions.

The first condition is caused by a widespread bacterial infection in the body called sepsis. The rash that may be present with this condition appears as pinpoint red dots all over the body. There is a simple way to test whether a red rash is the result of sepsis. If you press your finger against these red dots, they will not temporarily turn white, as most other rashes tend to do. Occasionally, you may also notice larger red or purple blotches along with these small pinpoint red dots. These are signs of a very dangerous infection, and you need to bring your baby to a medical facility immediately.

The other condition is caused by the transmission of genital herpes from the mother to the baby during delivery. This type of rash appears as clusters of white or yellowish blisters. The individual blisters are small, and they may pop in a few days. They may occur anywhere on the body, but they are especially concerning when they are located on the head or the face.

If you notice a rash that fits these descriptions, contact your doctor immediately. This is especially important if your baby is not feeding well, which could mean that the infection has spread to the brain or all over the body.

Roseola

Roseola is a common childhood rash that is caused by a type of herpes virus. Fortunately, this type of herpes virus is not the same as the ones that can cause serious infection of the brain. Unlike the other type of herpes virus, it is not a sexually transmitted infection and it does not cause genital herpes.

Infants between the ages of six months and a year old are most likely to get roseola. The infection typically causes a high fever and a rash. The rash of roseola is often described as small red dots, but they are usually not pinpoint in size. While the appearance of the rash can vary quite a bit in different individuals, it generally occurs all over the body, including the face.

Fortunately, roseola is not a dangerous infection. All it causes is fever and rash. The fever always precedes the rash, which lasts about three to four days. As soon as the fever goes away, the rash appears. Once the rash manifests itself, the fever should not return. The rash should resolve in two to three days as well. There is no known complication from this infection, aside from issues that are related to a high fever itself (as described on pages 55–57).

Besides fever control, there is no specific treatment for roseola. Since it is caused by a virus, antibiotics have no role in its management. If the fever lasts more than four days, or comes back after the rash appears, your child should be seen by a physician.

Jaundice

Jaundice is when an overabundance of a yellow pigment accumulates under the skin, resulting in a yellowish hue. Many babies become jaundiced, especially those of Asian descent.

This is usually a harmless condition, unless the level of jaundice becomes too high.

The yellow pigment is a waste product of broken-down blood cells. Babies are likely to have a higher level of this pigment because at birth they have a disproportionately high number of blood cells in their bodies. After birth, the baby's body starts to break down these excessive blood cells, and the pigment begins to accumulate as a by-product.

This by-product needs to be processed by the liver before it can be eliminated from the body. Unfortunately, an infant's liver is not as active as an adult's, and infants consequently cannot process the by-product pigment as fast as an adult would. The yellow pigment therefore piles up in the body and gets distributed to all the organs, including the skin.

Under normal circumstances, the body tolerates a low level of this yellow pigment. However, as the pigment level builds up, it can have detrimental effects on some organs, primarily the brain. If an excessive amount of the pigment gets stuck in the brain, it can lead to permanent brain damage. This type of disability can be devastating and may include hearing loss and the inability to walk.

 Essential

Older infants who consume a lot of vegetables, particularly carrots and sweet potatoes, may gain a yellow-orange tinge to their skins. This is not the same as jaundice, and it is a perfectly benign condition. You can distinguish this from jaundice by looking at the color of the white parts of the eyes. In true jaundice, the eyes become yellow along with the skin.

If you notice that your newborn baby's skin is yellow and his bilirubin level has not been determined in the past two or three days (a test that is normally performed in the hospital), you need to contact your pediatrician. This is particularly important if your baby's bilirubin level has never been evaluated. Sometimes if the initial bilirubin level is determined to be within a safe range, it may not be necessary to recheck it until a few days later. After the first week of life, the risk of jaundice is significantly lower.

Some people believe that breastfeeding makes jaundice worse. As long as the breastfeeding baby is ingesting an adequate amount of breast milk, this is not the case. In some situations, such as that when the baby has a hard time latching onto the nipple and maintaining suction, inadequate breastfeeding may contribute to a higher degree of jaundice. If your baby is not breastfeeding with enough frequency and duration, and if he has significant jaundice, you should consult your doctor about whether it is better to pump the breast milk out and feed your baby through a bottle.

Most importantly, parents must monitor their baby closely for increased yellowing of the skin. Make sure you observe the skin under natural indirect sunlight, as an artificial light source might exaggerate the yellowness of the skin. If the baby appears more and more yellow, you should contact your doctor without delay. The doctor might check the baby's blood to measure the exact level of the pigment in the body.

Red Spots All Over

About one in three babies develop a peculiar rash during the first week after birth. The rash first appears a day or two after birth, and it starts out as small pimples with a yellowish head in the center of each red spot. The rash can be quite extensive, in some cases covering almost the entire body.

Luckily, this entirely benign condition does not require any medical intervention. It's neither an allergic reaction nor a type of infection. This rash causes no discomfort to the baby, and after a week or so it fades away on its own.

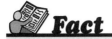 **Fact**

> The medical term for this rash is erythema toxicum. Despite its ominous-sounding name, this is a harmless condition that resolves spontaneously in a week or two. Doctors do not recommend applying any topical medication for this rash. There is no known medication that can hasten its resolution.

Diaper Rash

Virtually all babies end up with a diaper rash at one time or another. No matter how frequently you change your baby's diaper, the very fact that she wears one makes her susceptible to diaper rash.

Not all diaper rashes are created equal, however. Rashes typically start when the baby's ultrasensitive skin reacts to moisture in the diaper. This type of rash appears as an indistinct spread-out redness over areas of the skin covered by the diaper. It typically resolves with topical barrier creams and ointment designed to treat diaper rash.

Another type of diaper rash is caused by a common form of yeast that grows in the moist environment of the diaper. This rash appears as small, raised red dots, usually in the moist part of the skin covered by the diaper. Some of the dots can be fused with adjacent dots, forming one continuous patch of redness. The redness is usually significantly more intense than the typical non-yeast diaper rash.

The diaper rash that is caused by yeast does not respond to most over-the-counter medications. However, it does improve quickly with a prescribed antifungal cream or ointment. If you are not sure which type of diaper rash is afflicting your baby, consult your doctor—especially if a diaper rash fails to improve after using medication for more than a few days.

The Bellybutton

Newborns usually go home with the umbilical cord stump still attached to the body, and many parents feel unsure about how to take care of such a strange object. This section describes what to expect to happen with the umbilical stump and how to take care of it.

Care of the Stump

Some parents are apprehensive when it comes to taking care of their baby's umbilical stump. It appears gelatinous and soft at first, but it shrivels up in time. Hospital staff usually advises new parents to clean the stump with alcohol at every diaper change (or several times a day). However, some parents approach the bellybutton too gingerly, and the attachment doesn't get cleaned enough. As a result, the umbilical stump remains attached for a long time, sometimes longer than a month.

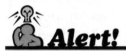

Alert!

If the skin surrounding the bellybutton becomes swollen and red, you need to contact your doctor right away. This could mean an infection of the bellybutton, a serious condition that requires antibiotic treatment.

If you clean it frequently and thoroughly with alcohol, the stump should fall off in two to three weeks. It's perfectly normal if it falls off sooner.

Something Smells Funny

Before the umbilical cord detaches, the tissue dies off gradually. Though this is a natural process, it can smell a little funny. It is not an indication of infection. In fact, there might even be a small amount of yellowish discharge from the stump. As long as the skin surrounding the bellybutton appears normal (that is, there is no redness, no swelling), you do not have to worry about an infection. Cleaning the stump frequently with alcohol-soaked cotton balls will also help with the smell. Even after the umbilical stump falls off, the smell may persist for some time. This is nothing to be concerned about as long as the skin around the bellybutton does not become red or swollen.

Spitting Up

Virtually all babies have spit-up episodes at one time or another; the question is when and whether you should be worried about it. Most babies spit up because the muscular valve-like structure in their stomach does not seal up very tightly as the stomach churns. It's analogous to shaking a bag full of fluid without sealing off the bag—some spillage is inevitable.

However, if your baby has projectile vomiting—that is, the spit-up literally flies across the room—another condition might be causing the vomiting. This type of forceful vomiting is very different from the typical spit-ups, not only in its strength but in the consistency of the spit-up. Projectile vomiting may indicate the presence of pyloric stenosis, a condition in which the milk cannot travel past the stomach and into the intestine. It generally occurs in babies between the ages of two weeks and two months and is quite rare after six months of age. If your baby consistently spits up with great projectile force after feeding, your doctor needs to examine her for pyloric stenosis.

Furthermore, if there is any trace of blood in the spit-up or in the stool, you need to contact your doctor. This may be a sign of food allergy. Some babies are allergic to the protein in cow's milk, which is the type of protein in most commercial formulas. Consult your doctor about whether you need to switch to a different type of formula.

Dealing with Croup

Croup is another common childhood infection that tends to affect older children more than newborns. However, when a young baby comes down with croup, the condition is more serious. Croup is caused by a virus that is somewhat related to the flu virus. Just as with the flu, children with croup also have fever and a severe cough.

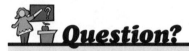 **Question?**

How can I tell if my child has croup or the flu?
The cough associated with croup typically has a very distinct quality—it is "barky," and your child may sound like a seal when coughing. However, not all children develop the characteristic barky cough, and the fever associated with croup can last just as long as a fever caused by the flu virus.

If you have an infant younger than six months who has a barky cough, it is important for his pediatrician to evaluate him for other respiratory problems. Croup can lead to a bacterial pneumonia secondarily, which is usually manifested when the fever fails to resolve after four days or with a worsening of the cough. If your child is older than two years, it is reasonable to administer over-the-counter cough suppressant to relieve the symptoms. If the cough lasts for more than two weeks, your pediatrician should evaluate your child.

Since croup is caused by a virus, antibiotics are useless against it. But if there is evidence of pneumonia, the use of antibiotics may be necessary.

CHAPTER 3

The Colic Dilemma

Colic is perhaps the most frustrating condition in all of pediatrics. Certainly, it is the source of tremendous anxiety for the parents of the estimated million babies in the United States who suffer from this condition. Driven by desperation, these parents go to great length in seeking a solution to stop their baby from crying. At best, these folk remedies and treatments do nothing to help the crying baby; at worst, they actually cause significant harm to the baby. It is paramount to separate the facts from the fiction when taking care of your colicky baby.

What Is Colic?

Colic is well known to most parents, yet it's a topic that's shrouded with misconceptions and fear. An encounter with parents of a colicky baby can be quite emotionally charged. By the time the baby makes it to the pediatrician's office, the parents have already suffered countless hours of a highly stressful situation. They want (and frequently need) a solution as soon as possible.

Crying for No Apparent Reason

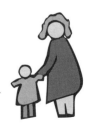

Medically, colic has a pretty exact definition. According to most medical textbooks, colic is when an infant less than six months old cries for more than ninety minutes a day. This might occur during a certain part of the day, with the early evening being most common. Since babies have no other mean of communicating, crying is their only way to express their needs and wants to the parents. All babies cry at one time or another, but when the crying becomes excessive compared to most other babies of the same age, health professionals call the condition colic.

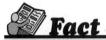 **Fact**

Most parents associate colic with gas or constipation, but the truth is that there is absolutely no relationship between colic and the intestinal system. Colic is completely unrelated to the abdomen, even though your baby is likely to expel a lot of gas during a colicky spell. The passing of the gas is a result of forceful crying rather than the cause.

One inherent criterion for the colic diagnosis is that the baby must be completely healthy. Excessive crying caused by an infection or an injury does not qualify as colic. Colic is crying for no apparent reason. The key word here is "apparent." All colicky babies cry for some reason, but with even the most advanced medical diagnostics, doctors cannot always determine the exact cause.

Of course, most parents have checked the obvious things by the time they seek medical attention. If your baby cries, you should first make sure that she is not hungry, that her diaper is not soiled or wet, and that she is not too hot or too cold. If you have gone through the list and eliminated the most common reasons for crying, and you still cannot ascertain why your baby is screaming, your baby may have colic.

No Pain
First off, it is important to clear up the most entrenched belief that colic is caused by pain. Most people believe this because

when a colicky baby cries, he sounds as if he is being tortured. This is not a weak cry but a vigorous and blood-curdling scream. The characteristic colic cry stands out from all other types of crying, such as that due to hunger or a dirty diaper.

While pediatric experts still cannot agree on the exact cause of colic, the consensus is that it is not a result of pain. It makes intuitive sense that colic is not a painful experience because none of the numerous methods used to calm a colicky baby involve giving pain reducers. In fact, medications frequently used for pain relief have no effect on the colicky baby.

It is a great relief for parents to learn that colic is not painful. Most assume that if their baby is crying that hard, he must be in a world of pain. Parents are happy to hear that their baby isn't suffering after all.

Danger Signs

Sometimes excessive crying without an apparent reason is actually an early indication of a serious medical condition. You need to know what to look for in case your baby is actually suffering from an illness.

Colic rarely starts right at birth. In fact, if your baby's excessive crying starts from day one, it is most likely that it is caused by something other than colic.

Most colicky babies start crying around two to four weeks after birth. The baby may be peaceful during the first few weeks of life, but then all of a sudden the sweet baby turns into a screaming horror. This sudden change is often a source of alarm for parents, even though this is the typical pattern of onset for colic.

Poor Feeding

If your baby stops feeding regularly or breaks away from the routine feeding schedule, you should be concerned. This is often an indication of a serious underlying medical problem. Colicky infants often have a vigorous suck and a voracious appetite. A healthy baby always has a good appetite—even a colicky one. If the feeding drops off, you need to have your baby examined by a physician.

Vomiting

Recurrent vomiting that is more than the typical spit-up is also a worrisome sign. Colicky babies occasionally throw up from vigorous crying, but this shouldn't happen repeatedly. If your baby throws up significantly more than usual, contact your pediatrician.

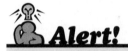

Alert!

Child abuse by another caregiver can manifest itself as vomiting and excessive crying in a baby. Serious internal injuries can be present without showing any external signs. Most commonly, internal head injuries or abdominal injuries can make the baby cranky without apparent reason.

Needless to say, if you find traces of blood in the spit-up, your baby needs to be seen by a health professional. Also, if the baby's vomit is mostly green, you have to contact your pediatrician. Throwing up green stuff could mean the presence of an intestinal blockage, which is a surgical emergency.

Hair Tourniquet

When a strand of hair wraps itself tightly around a finger, a toe, or even the penis, this can cause excruciating pain to the baby. Examine all the toes, fingers, and the penis of your boy baby to ensure that a hair tourniquet is not the reason for your baby's crying. Your pediatrician will also conduct a thorough head-to-toe examination when evaluating your baby for colic.

Corneal Abrasion

Sometimes a hard object can accidentally scratch the surface of your baby's eye. This can be quite painful for the baby, and the affected eye is often very teary. You cannot usually see the scratch on the eyeball yourself, but an eye specialist can detect such a scratch. If you suspect this may be the reason for your baby's crying, make an appointment with your doctor.

Fast Beats

Babies born with heart defects or irregular heartbeats can cry excessively when they experience extremely fast heartbeats. Even though infants usually tolerate fast heart rates better than older children, it is nevertheless very uncomfortable for them. They can appear cranky and refuse to feed well.

Children normally have a faster heart rate than adults, but the heart should not beat more than 180 times a minute when your child is at rest. Put your ear against your baby's chest and count the heart beats for thirty seconds. If you count more than 100 heartbeats in that time, you should have your baby checked by the doctor immediately.

Food Allergies Are Not to Blame

Parents can be quick to blame colic on a food allergy. Since babies less than four months old consume nothing but milk (either breast milk or formula), infant formula automatically becomes the culprit. However, there is plenty of scientific evidence that refutes this hypothesis.

Infant Formula as Scapegoat

Some people blame commercial infant formulas for causing colic. They attribute their baby's crying to discomfort caused by difficult-to-digest milk protein in the formula. Doctors know this is not the trigger for colic because switching formulas almost never stops a colicky baby from crying.

If your baby truly has milk protein allergy, she will most likely experience other problems, such as blood in the stool, extremely foul-smelling stools, or excessive vomiting. A colicky baby should not have these symptoms.

Breastfeeding Qualms

In addition, some mothers tend to blame themselves for the excessive crying that characterizes colic. They believe that there must be something in their diet that is showing up in their breast milk, thereby causing the baby to be fussy. In the vast majority of cases, this is untrue. There are very few foods in a breastfeeding mother's diet that will alter a baby's behavior.

While it is true that the food the mother ingests can alter the makeup and flavor of breast milk, these changes should not cause discomfort in babies. Most babies can taste the small trace amount of foods in the mother's diet, and they may feed less if they are not accustomed to the taste. However, it should not trigger crying or gas.

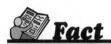 **Fact**

Dairy products in the mother's diet seldom cause stomach problems in babies, contrary to what many people claim. In addition, lactose intolerance in babies is an extremely rare condition. It is almost never the reason for your infant's excessive crying.

The few exceptions to this rule include alcohol and caffeine. The trace amount of alcohol that passes into breast milk can excessively sedate an infant. It is unclear whether this can be harmful to the baby and the developing brain, so most pediatricians recommend against alcohol consumption while breastfeeding.

Consumption of caffeinated drinks during breastfeeding can also affect your baby. She may take longer to fall asleep or may even act jittery. Be mindful of your caffeine intake while breastfeeding.

Is It Acid Reflux?

Reflux is an extremely common condition in babies. Adults frequently project their own experience onto their babies, but babies' stomachs are very different from those of adults. The acidity of an immature stomach is not nearly comparable to that of an adult's. Consequently, most babies do not experience discomfort when they have reflux problems.

Of course, there are some exceptions. Some babies do experience pain when they reflux. In fact, reflux issues are not necessarily accompanied by vomiting. When the food comes up, the baby simply tenses up her body and grimaces. Excessive crying can certainly occur with reflux, and this condition is sometimes misdiagnosed as colic.

It may sometimes be difficult to differentiate between reflux and colic, but there are a few helpful clues. The discomfort caused by reflux usually reaches its highest intensity within an hour after feeding. Thus, babies with reflux tend to cluster their crying after mealtime. A baby with true colic (without the reflux) is more likely to cry in the late afternoon or at night. Colicky babies cry most often when they are about to fall asleep, and the pattern does not correlate with their feeding schedule.

If you suspect your child might have reflux, get an appointment with your pediatrician. The doctor may prescribe a medication or order additional diagnostic tests to evaluate the reason for crying.

The True Cause of Colic

While there is no clear consensus on the cause of colic, most doctors agree that it has something to do with discomfort resulting from the baby's inability to regulate sleep. According to most experts who study colic, excessive crying may be a result of a baby's inability to easily transition between stages of the wake-sleep cycle.

The crying may occur as the baby is waking up or when the baby is trying to fall asleep. When the baby finds himself in this drowsy but not-quite-sleeping limbo, it's uncomfortable and frustrating. Many babies vent their steam by crying and screaming.

Currently, this is the most widely accepted theory of the cause of colic. Colic may very well have multiple causes, but scientists have not yet ascertained them.

Comforting Measures

There are plenty of things you can do to soothe your baby. While it may not be possible to prevent crying completely, the measures described in the following sections usually decrease the frequency as well as the duration of crying for your colicky baby.

A Bundle of Joy

Most babies prefer to be swaddled tightly when they're sleeping. This snug environment simulates the condition they became accustomed to inside the womb, so they feel secure and comforted when they are wrapped up in a tight bundle. But not all babies love swaddling. If your baby gets upset every time she's bundled up tightly, listen to her.

Some babies prefer to sleep in an infant car seat, the kind that unsnaps from its base and can be carried into the house by a handle. For them, it is the most comfortable place in the world. There is nothing wrong with having your baby strapped into the car seat while taking a nap. Just make sure that the car seat is placed on a sturdy surface and cannot fall.

Loud White Noise

Another way to comfort a colicky baby is to use a loud white noise. A constant machine-like noise is best for this purpose.

Many parents find out about this trick serendipitously when they are using the hair dryer or vacuuming the house. They notice that their colicky baby stops crying instantly when the motor starts running. Once the vacuum cleaner turns off, the crying resumes. It's almost as if there is an on-off switch for the baby's crying.

 Essential

It's hard to say exactly why colicky babies enjoy loud noises, but one theory is that the loud constant noise simulates the sound inside the womb. The constant sound of the mother's heartbeat, breathing, and blood rushing around in the body must be quite loud for the unborn child.

This white-noise trick usually works quite well, but you simply can't vacuum nonstop. Instead, there are commercial audio CDs that generate white noise for these babies. If you want, you can even record your own white noise album by taping the sound of vacuum cleaners and lawnmowers.

Good Vibration

A gentle vibration or motion can often comfort a colicky infant; perhaps the movement resembles the motion experienced inside the womb as the mother walked around. Parents can achieve this motion either with a bouncy chair that vibrates or a mechanical swing. Holding and rocking the baby may be even more effective, but you can't do that all day and all night.

Light at the End of the Tunnel

Most colicky babies stop their crying spells by the time they are around four months of age. This can vary somewhat, depending on the baby. It is very unusual for colic to last past six months of age. Even for the unfortunate parents who have to tolerate excessive crying for more than six months, there is *always* an end to the crying. Keep this fact in mind when you're dealing with a colicky infant. It may just be the saving grace that pulls you through the toughest days.

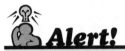

Alert!

No matter how frustrated you feel, never shake your baby. A baby's brain is extremely delicate. Violent shaking can permanently damage the brain, causing irreversible neurological deficit or even death. Before you become too frustrated, step away from the baby and take a break from it all.

Don't forget that your pediatrician is always available for counseling. You may frequently feel that you are at your wit's end when dealing with a colicky infant, and your doctor is a wonderful resource to alleviate your fears and frustration. If your baby has been crying for more than three hours, feel free to contact your pediatrician for advice.

CHAPTER 4

Growth and Development

One of the greatest joys of being a parent comes from watching your child thrive and mature from a helpless little baby to a thinking human being. During this process, your child will undoubtedly go through countless changes. Sometimes these changes occur gradually, but sometimes they are less subtle. Accompanying the process of metamorphosis, there are also innumerable myths and misconceptions along the way. Understanding child development allows you to be alert when something unexpected happens.

Growing Concerns

All pediatricians document their patients' growth in a standard growth chart. It is one of the best ways to evaluate the overall health of a child. It is equally important for parents to know how to interpret the numbers derived from a growth chart. Most pediatricians assume that parents inherently have the knowledge to read a growth chart, but this assumption doesn't always match up to reality.

Pediatricians often refer to the absolute measurements, such as ounces and pounds for your child's weight, and inches or centimeters for height, length, and head circumference. Pediatricians also track the percentile of these measurements. The absolute measurements are straightforward enough,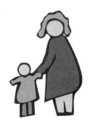

even though they deserve a brief discussion. The percentile of growth requires a more lengthy discussion.

Growth Charts

The best way to explain the percentile of growth indicated by the growth chart is to use an example. If your child is in the 25th percentile along the curve for height, it does not mean that his height is only one quarter of an average child's height. Instead, it means that he is taller than 25 percent of his peers who are the same age. He is shorter than the remaining 75 percent of children his age.

 Essential

There is no reason to be alarmed if your child's growth percentile seems to fluctuate up and down at different ages. Unless there's a steady and persistent slowing or acceleration, this type of fluctuation is expected for normal growth. Children go through growth spurts, and children often go up and down on the percentile curve during the growing years.

If your child plots out very low on the growth curve, it doesn't necessarily mean that there is something wrong with him. Just like adults, healthy children come in all shapes and forms. If your child stays low on the growth curve but nevertheless gains weight steadily at the same rate as other children, most pediatricians will not be alarmed by this growth pattern. On the other hand, if your child starts out around the 95th percentile and suddenly drops down to the 10th percentile in a short period of time, there is usually something wrong. Even if he gains weight and height, the rate of growth may be too slow to be considered normal.

If a sudden slowing in growth occurs, your pediatrician will take a detailed history of your child's total food intake. There are many conditions that can trigger a deceleration of growth, and additional blood tests may be necessary to ascertain the cause.

Head Circumference

Pediatricians monitor your baby's head circumference from birth to three years. It is measured with a tape to find out the greatest circumference of the head just above the ears. After three years of age, the growth of the head does not have much clinical significance.

If the size of a child's head increases too slowly, it could indicate a problem with her brain development. In this case, the brain might not be developing as fast as it should. On the other hand, if the head expands too rapidly, it could mean that something is obstructing the flow of fluid inside the brain. This could be an early sign of a brain tumor. Unlike weight and height, more is not necessarily better when it comes to your baby's head circumference.

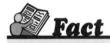 **Fact**

One of the most common reasons for your baby to have a large head is familial macrocephaly. This means that big heads are inherited, and it doesn't necessarily mean that something is wrong. If a child's parents have large heads, the baby is more than likely going to have a large head circumference as well.

Your pediatrician will alert you if your child's head size is abnormal, and the next step in evaluation depends on other clinical findings.

Developmental Milestones

At each well-baby visit, your pediatrician will ask you whether you have any specific concerns about your baby's development. She will also ask whether your baby has begun to do certain things by certain ages, such as tracking your movements with his eyes or reacting playfully to your hand motions. A delay in attaining certain motor skills can be the earliest sign of cerebral palsy, which results from a dysfunction or damage in the brain. Early detection of neurological conditions like this is paramount in developing children, because delay in treatment can adversely affect the quality of life for these children as adults.

While most parents are not experts in child development, they usually have a fairly good sense of what to expect in terms of their baby's ability to do certain things. However, there are some common misconceptions about developmental milestones that need to be clarified.

Rolling Over

Many babies surprise their parents by mastering the art of rolling over at a very early age. Even though most babies cannot roll over until after four months of age, some precocious infants manage to do so before the age of two months.

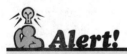

Alert!

Always be wary of where you leave your infant. Many early-rolling babies suffer falls from heights, such as a bed or changing table, because their parents weren't expecting them to roll around yet. Always have one hand on the baby when you are changing diapers. You never know when she's going to surprise you by turning over for the first time.

On the other hand, some babies cannot roll over until after six months of age. If this is the case with your child, ask your pediatrician to pay close attention to your child's motor development and muscle tone. There is usually no reason to be alarmed, but extra vigilance never hurts.

Crawling

Babies generally start crawling between the ages of six and ten months. While most babies learn how to crawl before they manage to take their first walking step, some babies completely skip the developmental milestone of crawling. One day out of the blue, they simply take off and go from sitting to walking. If your baby does not crawl by a certain age, there is usually no need to be worried. Ask your pediatrician, if you are still concerned.

For those babies who do crawl, this motor skill poses additional risk to the infant. New safety concerns arise with the attainment of mobility for the baby. Parents and other care providers must stay vigilant at all times after a baby learns how to crawl.

Even though most babies crawl on all fours, innovative babies may also think outside the box. They often scoot backward, pivot on one arm and one leg to move forward, or drag their feet behind them as they claw their way around. There is no right way to crawl. As long as it gets the child from point A to point B efficiently, parents do not need to intervene or correct the crawling style.

Walking

For most parents, this is one of the big monumental milestones in their baby's life. Taking the first step is an exciting moment for the baby as well as the parents, and the baby seems to realize this. He laughs nervously as he stretches out his leg and makes this giant leap in his developmental history. With each successful step, he rejoices and feels tremendously proud of his newfound independence.

 Essential

It is unnecessary to buy shoes for your child when she first starts walking. In fact, walking barefoot may help strength the muscles in the feet and help her gain better balance during the first few months of walking. Shoes are only designed to protect the feet from rough walking surfaces. There is no need for them if your toddler is just going to run around indoors.

However, when the fireworks finish and the dust settles, parents suddenly realize the meaning of their baby's mobility. All the places in the house that used to be unreachable for their child now potentially threaten the toddler with the possibility of cuts and bruises. Hopefully, you have already childproofed your house by this time.

Behavioral Problems

As your young child grows and acquires new skills, not everything she learns will be positive. There is no shortage around your child of bad examples from bad-behaving older children and even adults to give her ideas. It is the responsibility of all parents to recognize this bad behavior and correct it as early as possible before it becomes a bad habit.

Biting

Children bite for many reasons. Some infants are simply exploring their world with their new teeth. There is no malicious intent behind these bites. When a young infant bites, the parent is encouraged to immediately pull the infant away from the bitten body part. The goal is to send a clear signal that such behavior is unacceptable.

Older children who bite out of frustration need much stronger deterrent for their act. A clear message must be sent as soon as the biting occurs that such behavior is not tolerated. For children older than two, some forms of discipline should be instituted right away after such incident occurs. A time-out chair would be an appropriate option.

Thumb Sucking and Nail Biting

Thumb sucking and nail biting are a couple of behaviors that usually defy any attempt at curtailment. Pediatricians and developmental experts have no reliable way of stopping either behavior. Unfortunately, both of these habits can increase your child's risk of getting an infection due to the prolonged hand-to-mouth contact. The only thing pediatricians can offer is to remind parents that most children eventually stop sucking their thumbs. Alas, the same thing cannot be said for nail-biters. Many of them grow up to be mature and highly skilled nail-biting adults.

A Matter of Speaking

The ability to speak is one of the most important skills a child can acquire. In fact, speech is the distinctive characteristic that sets human beings apart from the animals. When a child encounters difficulties in this process, the parents naturally become concerned. Your child's future depends on his success in mastering the art of communication.

Speech Delay

Most children utter their first recognizable word before they turn a year old, though some children are late bloomers. Generally speaking, pediatricians do not get overly concerned until a child fails to use any word after eighteen months. This is usually the threshold for doctors to refer a child to audiology to evaluate his hearing. Beside hearing impairment, other conditions, including autism and mental retardation, can also delay speech. After the pediatrician sets the investigation into motion, a panel of experts usually assesses the child with speech delay to ascertain the cause.

Some children have no problem using words, but their speech is often difficult to understand to people outside the family. This difficulty with articulation is called a lisp. During the acquisition of speech, all normal and otherwise healthy children can develop a lisp at one time or another. This is not a concern unless this pattern of speech causes embarrassment or anxiety for the child. Talk to your pediatrician if you are worried about your child's lisping.

Stuttering

Stuttering is characterized by a speech that is lacking in fluency. The flow of the words is often interrupted by pauses, repetition of syllables or words, or drawn-out vowel sounds. Disruption in fluency is common for children starting to learn to speak, typically from age two to six. It is considered normal until it causes undue tension and embarrassment to the child.

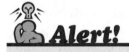

Alert!

Parents of stuttering children need to be patient. It is paramount for you to provide a relaxing home environment for your child to practice speech in a safe condition. Never blame or criticize a child for a halting speech. Such negative feedback can only intensify anxiety and worsen stuttering.

Fortunately, most children outgrow their stuttering, and less than 1 percent of adults stutter. For those who are plagued by stuttering into older childhood, an early consultation with a speech therapist is recommended. In addition, a supportive family is extremely important in helping children overcome this problem. Do not hurry a stuttering child to finish the sentence. External pressure tends to worsen stuttering. Allow plenty of time for the child to finish his sentence. Avoid finishing the thought for him. Most importantly, make every speaking opportunity as relaxing as possible.

Bedwetting

Parents may not consider bedwetting a childhood illness, but it is nevertheless a medical condition that can cause significant psychological trauma for a child. It is no less serious than any other chronic medical condition. It deserves to be brought to the attention of the pediatrician because treatment options do exist for this condition.

Avoid Blame

Since no one is born with voluntary bladder control, it is a universal and normal condition for a child to bed wet until she becomes potty trained. Most pediatricians do not consider it to be a problem until the child reaches the age of six or seven. Even though it is extremely common, it can be a source of embarrassment and tension in the family. When dealing with this issue, it is essential not to blame your child when there has been an accident in bed. In all likelihood, she is embarrassed enough already about what happened.

When accidents happen, take a deep breath and relax. You may be somewhat upset by the prospect of having to change the sheets for the fourth time in a week, but you should not make the task of cleaning up your first priority. Instead, the first thing you should do is to comfort your child and reassure her that it is okay and she has not done anything wrong. Most of all, it is important to remember that bedwetting is a self-limiting problem. It is going to go away, sooner or later. When it may happen is tricky to determine for each individual, but it generally becomes less common as the child gets older. Most children grow out of this problem by age fifteen.

Even though it may seem like a lost cause at first, there are actually many things you can do to minimize the frequency of bedwetting.

Change the Nighttime Routine

First of all, your child should not drink any type of fluid in the two hours prior to bedtime. This rule may be impractical to follow since suppertime falls late for many families, but try your best to adhere to this schedule. It goes a long way in lessening the frustration and saving time laundering sheets. If the child is thirsty and begs for something to drink, it is okay for him to chew some ice chips or take a small sip of water prior to going to sleep. But don't allow this little exception to be abused. If your child asks repeatedly for something to drink, you have to put your foot down and request that he go to bed. Once is reasonable; twice is a sign that your child may be trying to take advantage of the system.

Secondly, limit your child's consumption of caffeinated drinks. Ideally, children should not have any soda or tea at all, but if it is a special occasion, they can have a moderate amount of these drinks during the day. Caffeine is a powerful diuretic. It directly stimulates the kidneys to produce more urine.

Finally, you should incorporate visiting the potty just prior to going to bed as part of the bedtime ritual. This at least ensures an empty bladder at the beginning of sleep, and hopefully translates into a dry night. In fact, this is a good idea not only for children with a bedwetting problem but for every member of the family. If everyone empties his bladder prior to retiring, the bedwetting child won't feel that he is being singled out.

Some experts suggest that a parent wake the child up in the middle of the night and take him to the potty. Though this might curtail some incidences of bedwetting, many pediatricians believe it is too disruptive, for both the parent and the child. If you don't mind waking up on a regular basis, you could try this method to see how well it works for your child.

Bells and Whistles

If fluid restriction and bedtime voiding do not help your child with the bedwetting problem, another effective means of curtailing this habit is the use of specialized electronic alarms. These alarms have a sensor that is secured to your child's underwear and a small speaker that emits an audible alert when the sensor detects moisture.

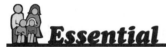

Essential

Pediatricians recommend a medical evaluation to rule out possible urinary-tract infection or kidney problems for any child who still experience bedwetting after the age of six. The investigation usually involves a brief interview followed by a physical examination and a quick analysis of your child's urine specimen. Invasive and painful blood tests are usually unnecessary.

When the alarm goes off, your child may or may not wake up. It is the parent's job to wake the child and lead him to the bathroom to use the toilet. The process of training your child to respond to the alarm may take quite a long time, but it is generally effective for many bedwetters. Be patient, as it can take as long as eight to sixteen weeks before your child can wake up on his own and eventually stop wetting the bed altogether. More than half of the children who are rid of their bedwetting do not experience any relapse of the problem after they master control of their bladders. Nevertheless, the alarm is not universally successful. If it does not work for your child, there are other options to pursue.

The Role of Medication

Not all parents feel comfortable with the idea of altering their child's hormone level to control bedwetting. It's perfectly fine if you are reluctant to try this approach, but many parents swear by it and it has brought happiness and salvation to their households. It is an option that should be at least considered if all else has failed.

Before you dismiss the possibility of using these medications, keep in mind that they are safe and nonaddictive. At the same time, is not typically recommended that they be taken on a daily basis. They are generally prescribed for use only on special occasions, like a pajama party or sleepover at a friend's house. Used in the short term and episodically, they are extremely effective.

The medication is called DDAVP, or desmopressin. This medication is a chemical that is very similar to the natural hormones synthesized by the brain to regulate urine production. It comes in a liquid form, which is sprayed in the nose, or in a tablet form.

Unlike the older generation of medications for bedwetting, DDAVP is safer and has fewer side effects. It might cause a mild stomach upset and headache in some children, but this is not common. Even though it works quite well on a short-term basis, its effect tends to wear off after chronic use. After a week or two, the dose must be increased for the medication to maintain its efficacy. Because children's bodies generally get used to the medicine fairly quickly, most pediatricians recommend using this medication for temporary relief only.

CHAPTER 5

The Fever Fear

A s a universal reaction to a variety of conditions, fever is ubiquitous. It can often assist the body in the process of recovery. However, it is often a source of great anxiety for parents because they fear that the fever itself may cause harm to the child. This chapter discusses the various causes for fever and how to manage them in specific situations. It will allay some of your concerns and allow you to make better decisions when your child has a fever.

What Is a Fever?

Fever is one of the most common reasons for parents to bring their children in for a doctor's visit. Parents tend to worry less about a headache, diarrhea, or even a fracture than a high fever. Regardless of cultural background or socioeconomic level, parents worry that their children might suffer brain damage caused by high temperature. However, virtually all doctors know that an elevated temperature induced by a viral infection never causes injury to the brain. Instead, it is the underlying infection that sometimes damages the brain. As long as the fever is caused by a minor viral infection, it is unnecessary to obsessively worry about the high temperature itself. (As stated in Chapter 2, however, any fever is potentially dangerous for children under the age of two months. A child of this age who experiences a fever should be taken to the pediatrician.)

What Causes Fever?

Fever is usually a normal response to a state of inflammation in the body. For children, the most common causes of fever are viral infections and minor bacterial infections, with viral infections causing the majority of fevers. This is a good thing, because the vast majority of children get better on their own without suffering long-term disabilities or complications.

Bodies generate a fever to shorten the duration of the infection. At an elevated temperature, the immune system works faster and more effectively. In short, the fever is created by the body and not by the invading viruses or germs. It makes inherent sense, then, that the body would not do something to harm itself. Therefore, under most circumstances fevers are harmless.

What Is Normal Body Temperature?

This sounds like a straightforward question that everyone should be able to answer, but many parents worry themselves sick about a slightly elevated temperature that may not be a fever at all. To understand fever, you must first understand the normal range of human body temperatures.

A lot of people believe any temperature that is higher than 98.6°F is a fever. However, most medical professionals agree that a fever is any properly measured body temperature that is at or higher than 100.4°F. Anything lower than that is not considered a fever at all. Even a fever of 100.4°F or higher is considered a very slight temperature (or low-grade temperature, as doctors call it). A moderate temperature is one that is higher than 102.2°F, and a high temperature is anything more than 104°F.

A healthy child's body temperature fluctuates throughout the day. The body's temperature tends to drop to its lowest in the middle of the night, and it rises to its peak in the late afternoon. In addition, the body's temperature can be affected by a child's emotional state, activity level, and even environmental conditions. Not taking this variation into consideration when interpreting a temperature is a common mistake that many parents make.

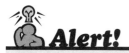

Alert!

It's not uncommon for parents to resort to desperate and drastic cooling measures in an attempt to reduce a child's body temperature. But some of these practices have been proven unsafe and can pose a serious health hazard to the child.

More importantly, the exact degree of the child's temperature is less significant than how long the fever lasts and how the child looks. Taking a child's temperature may clue you in as to whether your child has a fever, but it does not give you any clues about what might be causing the fever—nor does it provide any information on the severity of the illness.

How High Is Too High?

One of the questions parents most frequently ask is, "How high does the temperature have to get before I should bring my child to the emergency room?" This question implies that when the temperature is too high, bodily harm will occur. This is, however, generally not true.

Under normal circumstances, a fever generated by the body itself (that is, not by a super-heated external environment) does not raise the child's temperature above 107°F. Experienced pediatricians rarely see children whose fever runs higher than 106°F. (While temperatures this high are uncommon, they are definitely not unheard of.)

Most children who run a fever have a cold or other viral infection, and they generally recover uneventfully. In other words, a high fever does not necessarily mean someone has a bacterial infection. The point is that the degree of the fever does not always correlate with the severity of the underlying illness.

It is true, however, that if a child's temperature rises above 107°F, the body is not likely to tolerate it well for very long. Fortunately, a body temperature above this level does not happen except in extraordinary circumstances, so most of the time, parents do not have to worry about temperature going out of control.

Fever caused by a cold or other viral infection usually does not rise above 102°F. If your child's temperature rises above that point and stays there without fluctuating for a period of time, you should visit your pediatrician.

Hot Headed

Another misconception that many parents have is that you can tell where the infection is located by simply locating the spot on the child's body where the temperature is hottest. A lot of parents say that they are particularly concerned because the head feels very hot to the touch compared to the rest of the body. They are worried because they think this pattern could indicate that there is an infection in the child's head. Similarly, if the belly feels very hot, they believe the infection must be lodged in the stomach.

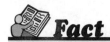 *Fact*

As the child's body temperature rises, the body naturally distributes most of the blood in the central parts of the body, thereby raising the temperature. The arms and legs tend to feel cold to the touch, and the head and body feel hotter. The surface temperature of these areas has nothing to do with the cause of the fever or where the illness is localized.

Unfortunately, there is no basis for this belief. Otherwise, it would be a lot easier to gauge the source of infections. When a child's head feels hot, it simply means that she could be running a fever. Having a hot head does not mean that the infection is inside the head or is more serious than heat perceived anywhere else on the body.

Fever in the Right Perspective

Parents and doctors often have very different views about fever. For something as ubiquitous as fever, this dichotomy often leads to all sorts of misunderstandings and anxieties. This section is intended to narrow the gap between these drastically different views and allow parents to understand their pediatrician's way of thinking.

The Origin of Fever Fear

There must be a historical explanation of why this fear of fever evolved in the first place. Many decades ago, before the advent of antibiotics, a high fever usually indicated the presence of an infection. Occasionally, those were bacterial infections that led to serious consequences, including fatality. With most viral infections, such as a cold, there usually isn't a high temperature that exceeds 102°F. This tendency of associating high fevers only with bacterial infections made people conclude that fever itself was the dangerous condition.

With the diagnostic capability of modern medicine and close follow-up with the doctor, it is generally not difficult to distinguish a bacterial infection from a viral one (with a few exceptions that will be specifically addressed later). As long as they are able to assure the absence of a serious bacterial infection, physicians are generally comfortable observing the patient closely without resorting to diagnostic tests.

The Physician's Take on Fever

On the other hand, this fear about fever isn't entirely unfounded. When body temperature gets very high (that is, more than 104°F), most physicians would be concerned. However, the doctor's concern is usually focused on what might be causing the fever rather than on the fever itself. Parents, on the other hand, tend to be more concerned about the direct effect of the fever rather than curious about what might be triggering it. This distinction cannot be repeated enough.

 Essential

The overall duration of a fever is much more significant than the actual temperature itself. In most cases, doctors start to worry about a fever if it has lasted more than four days, regardless of the cause.

The duration of a fever has much more clinical relevance than the fever's degree, as a temperature that lasts over many days may indicate that something more serious is evolving from the initial infection. A simple viral infection can sometimes weaken the body enough to allow bacteria to invade. When this happens, the initial fever might be prolonged, or the fever might abate and then return. Physicians are much more concerned with this fever pattern because the secondary bacterial infection could be much more serious than the initial viral one.

Many years of clinical observation have revealed that there is a genetic tendency to develop either high fevers or low ones, depending on the individual. Similar to the great variations in children's height and weight, there is also a wide distribution of temperatures when a child gets sick. Some individuals tend to run a high fever with virtually any infection, even a minor cold.

Fever and Complications

Fever is frequently associated with many other symptoms, and it is blamed for a variety of complications. Most of these beliefs are unsupported, but some of them may actually have some merit. For example, while high fevers do not trigger seizures in the vast majority of children, a sudden rise in temperature could cause seizure attacks in a small percentage of children (as discussed on pages 57–58).

The Teething Fever

Strangely enough, many health-care providers still believe that a child can get a fever while teething. Many members of this camp reason that since the gums are inflamed during teething, the degree of inflammation may trigger a fever. Many guidebooks written by pediatricians claim that there is such an association between fever and teething. However, none of these books cites any medical-journal research study that might provide evidence for such a claim.

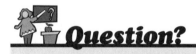 *Question?*

How can I be sure that teething doesn't cause fever?
Results from well-conducted medical research have shown that a temperature greater than 102°F is *never* associated with teething. If a fever is present, there must be some other cause, because teething is not the culprit.

Indeed, this correlation has been refuted by research performed in carefully controlled settings. There is no proven link between teething and fever. However, many of the other symptoms associated with teething are true, such as increased drooling, poor appetite, inclination to gnaw on things, and irritability. Still, fever is not one of those measurable symptoms. If you were to compare a child who is teething to one who is not, you would find that the teething child's body temperature was only slightly elevated (by no more than 1 degree), and the rise in temperature wasn't significant enough to be qualified as a fever.

Why then do so many babies develop a high temperature when they are teething? It's due to an unfortunate timing of developmental milestones. Most tooth eruptions occur between four months and fifteen months of age. Coincidentally, this is also the period of time when babies become more mobile and active. When babies finally learn how to sit up, crawl, and walk around, they immediately become susceptible to a much wider range of infections. As they explore the world, they touch everything around them. They also love putting their fingers and other objects into their mouths. This is the perfect way to catch a virus, and when they get sick from these viruses, they are more likely to develop a fever.

Fever-Induced Seizures

Many people believe that if a fever gets too high, it will invariably trigger a seizure. Pediatricians know that this is definitely not the case. It is true that some children are born with the tendency to have convulsions when their body temperature rises rapidly. However, this condition only applies to 4 percent of healthy children. Doctors call this condition febrile seizure. Even though the fever may be the trigger for the seizure, the fever itself doesn't cause the development of a tendency for seizures. A high temperature simply reveals the underlying propensity in a given child to develop seizures. The majority of children who do not suffer from febrile seizures will not have seizures, no matter how high their fever gets.

The likelihood that a child will have febrile seizures is partly determined by genetics. If either parent suffered from febrile seizures as a child, their baby will have a greater chance than the general population of developing this condition. (How much greater is hard to say, as the degree of heritability is difficult to quantify.) In addition, this tendency to have febrile seizures goes away after six years of age, so it is definitely not a life-long condition. Adults and older children never have febrile seizures.

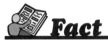 **Fact**

Only 4 percent of healthy children are likely to develop a seizure when their temperature goes up. This propensity for seizure goes away after six years of age. The likelihood for a child to have febrile seizures is inherited genetically.

Seizure Prevention

Most parents believe that seizures themselves cause permanent damage to the brain. As scary as it may be to witness your child going through a seizure, the seizure attack itself is rarely dangerous. If the seizure does not last more than a few minutes, it is virtually impossible for it to cause any harm to the brain. Even if a child ends up having a seizure that was triggered by a fever, there is no need to fret over the possibility of brain damage.

Most children will never have a seizure, no matter how high their fever runs. For those few children who do have the propensity to develop seizures, research has clearly shown that aggressive regimen of fever reducers does not prevent febrile seizures from recurring. The only proven method to prevent febrile seizures is a daily dose of antiseizure medication. Most physicians do not recommend this because of the potential serious side effects of taking an antiseizure medication on a long-term basis.

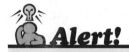

Alert!

It is not necessary to take your child to the emergency room every time she has a febrile seizure. If the seizure lasts less than a few minutes and does not recur, just call the pediatrician for an appointment.

What can a parent do for a child with a past history of febrile seizures? Most doctors recommend reducing the fever with medication. Even though this does not ward off potential seizures, lowering the temperature does make the child more comfortable. If a seizure occurs with the elevated temperature, it is advisable to lay the child down on his or her side. If the seizure lasts more than a few minutes, call the paramedics. If the seizure stops on its own after a few seconds, it's still a good idea to call the pediatrician and make an appointment. Each seizure should be communicated to the physician. If the seizures are frequent, other management options must be considered with the help of a pediatric neurologist.

When to Worry about a Fever

Even though most of this chapter is devoted to assuaging parents' fear of fevers, there are times when pediatricians are genuinely concerned about a fever. One of those times is when the infant is less than six weeks old.

Fever and Your Baby

The first six weeks for your baby is a special period in a child's life. Infants less than a month old have very weak immune systems. They do not have the same arsenal of defenses against infection as older children. To make matters worse, they often do not manifest infections in the same way as older children. Not only do they lack the ability to communicate, they cannot generate an effective fever at times. If an infant less than six weeks old has just a low-grade fever (temperature higher than 100.4°F), physicians usually take no chances and go all out to investigate a possible bacterial infection. This usually includes blood tests, urine tests, and a spinal tap to check for infection of the brain.

The reaction may seem drastic, but there is no room for guesswork when it comes to a baby with potential bacterial infection. The consequences of missing a serious infection can be devastating, and there is simply too much at stake.

Special Circumstances

Another group of patients that is the exception to the rule are children with deficient immune systems. This is a fairly large group that consists of patients with sickle cell disease, children with organ transplants who are taking immune-suppressing drugs, children with AIDS, children with immune-altering conditions such as lupus or juvenile arthritis, children with certain liver disorders and kidney diseases, children without spleens, and children with cancer. Parents of these children are often cautioned by their physicians about their child's fragile state in advance, and they typically know exactly what to do when their children get a fever.

In addition, patients with certain implanted devices should also take fever seriously. Many patients with chronic illnesses who have catheters implanted in their bodies need to worry about fever because these implants make it easier for infections to find their way into the bloodstream, and catheters tend to trap bacteria.

Prolonged Fever

If your child has a fever that has lasted for more than four days, you should go to the pediatrician. It is unusual for a fever to last this long if it is caused by a virus. Physicians in general do not worry about how high a fever gets but rather how long the fever lasts. Health professionals feel that a fever that lasts more than three to four days is cause for more concern. A prolonged fever almost always indicates the presence of a bacterial infection or other more serious conditions. Occasionally, a medication itself can trigger a fever, but this is more likely to happen in the hospital setting.

If your child has a prolonged fever that is associated with a stiff neck and headache, seek medical attention immediately. This combination of symptoms could mean that your child may have an infection in the brain.

Common Causes of Fever

Fever is the common denominator for a lot of childhood illnesses. As mentioned previously, autoimmune disorders, infections, or even a reaction to medication can trigger a fever. This section focuses on a few common causes of fever.

Roseola

Roseola is perhaps one of the most common causes of fever for children. The fever that is associated with roseola typically spikes suddenly, and it is usually very high (104°F is not uncommon). Despite the high fever, the child often appears comfortable and playful. The fever is frequently followed by an eruption of rash though this does not occur in everyone. It is entirely possible to have roseola with just the fever and with no rash at all. As with most fevers triggered by a viral infection, the duration of the fever is normally short (less than four days). Occasionally, it can last seven days, which would prompt most physicians to conduct investigative blood and urine tests.

Urinary Tract Infections

Urinary tract infections (UTIs) are the type of bacterial infection that most commonly requires hospitalization for children. Children younger than six months are routinely managed with inpatient care and intravenous antibiotics. The reason pediatricians treat urinary tract infections seriously is because if the infection spreads to the kidneys, permanent kidney damage can result. If the kidney infection is severe enough, kidney function may fail completely, requiring the patient to stay on dialysis indefinitely.

 ## Essential

Children over three years old can reliably report a painful sensation with urination when they have a UTI. Unfortunately, younger children cannot usually vocalize their discomfort. As a result, any child under the age of two with a high fever (greater than 101°F) without any apparent source for the fever needs to have her urine examined for evidence of infection.

If your toddler has a fever for more than three days but has no other symptoms (such as a runny nose, cough, vomiting, or diarrhea), you should bring him to the doctor's office to make sure there is no bacterial infection or UTI present. Keep in mind that before your child is potty-trained, the only way to obtain an urine specimen from him may be via catheterization of the bladder.

Mononucleosis

Mononucleosis, simply called "mono" by most people, is another viral infection that can cause a prolonged fever without any apparent source. Mononucleosis most commonly affects older children, adolescents, and even adults. People who come down with this infection usually feel extremely tired as well as feverish. Many have some degree of soreness in the throat during the initial phase of the infection, and most also have enlarged glands around the neck.

Scarlet Fever

Scarlet fever is nothing more than a strep throat run rampant. It used to be a life-threatening infection, but over the past century, the strain of bacteria that causes the infection has become significantly weaker. No one knows why this is so, but scarlet fever no longer causes death in children.

Scarlet fever usually starts out as a run-of-the-mill strep throat. Soreness in the throat, fever, and nasal congestion are common initial symptoms. However, when the toxin made by the strep bacteria spreads into the bloodstream, scarlet fever occurs.

The rash associated with scarlet fever is very rough. When you run your finger across the surface of the skin, it almost feels like sandpaper. The rest of the skin is typically very red, similar to a bad sunburn. The fever coexists with the rash, and a general sensation of fatigue is common.

If you suspect your child might have scarlet fever, you need to get an appointment with your doctor within a few days. Even though scarlet fever is no longer a lethal infection, untreated scarlet fever or strep throat can sometimes cause rheumatic fever or glomerulonephritis, conditions that occur when the immune system inappropriately attacks the heart or the kidneys, respectively.

Comforting a Fever

Even though a high temperature does not directly harm the body, it is nevertheless very uncomfortable for a child to have a fever. In addition, a prolonged fever can cause a child to become dehydrated and raise his or her metabolic needs, both of which can further weaken a sick child. You can still do a great deal to make your child more comfortable when he develops a fever.

Good Hydration Makes Sense

Drinking plenty of cool fluids is always a good idea for a child who has a fever. This is one of those pieces of ancient wisdom that has clear merits. When the body temperature rises, breathing becomes more rapid, and the skin gets flushed. Both of these reactions to fever hasten the rate at which the body loses water. More of the body's water is lost as vapor through breathing, and more moisture dissipates from the skin when the temperature is higher. Many children lose interest in drinking and eating while they run a fever, but it is important to constantly remind them to take in additional fluids to prevent dehydration. In addition, the child will feel better when he is well hydrated. It may be difficult to convince a sick child to drink water constantly, but it's well worth the effort.

Sugary drinks and Popsicles are not as good as pure water when it comes to keeping your child hydrated, but if they are the only things your child will take, they can be used as a last resort.

Other Cooling Measures

Besides drinking, additional cooling measures can be safely applied to the feverish child. A wet towel can be used to cool her off. Soak the towel with room-temperature water (not ice-cold water), and drape it over your child's shoulders. This not only brings her temperature down slightly, it can also make her feel a lot better. Applying a cool wet towel to your child's forehead also helps to lower her temperature, but draping the towel over her shoulders is generally more effective because it covers a larger body surface area for faster cooling.

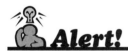

Alert!

Some parents advocate cooling the child's skin with cloths soaked with rubbing alcohol. This is a dangerous recommendation, as the skin can absorb some of the alcohol and cause serious intoxication or neurological problems. This practice is even more dangerous for young infants, as their skin absorbs chemicals faster than the skin of older children and adults. This practice should always be avoided.

Using ice-cold water is not recommended because it simply causes too much discomfort to the child. In addition, if the cold water causes the child to shiver, it can actually elevate a body temperature that is already high. Shivering causes the muscles to contract, and these frequent involuntary contractions can raise the body temperature even more. Imagine someone dumping ice water on you when you're already shivering—it's extremely unpleasant.

Using Fever Reducers

Fever reducers are very useful medications in lowering the body temperature and making your child feel better. The most common fever-reducing agents for children are acetaminophen (commonly known as Tylenol) and ibuprofen (commonly known as Motrin or Advil). These medications work in different ways to lower body temperature. The effect of acetaminophen lasts for three to four hours, and the effect of ibuprofen lasts longer, generally five to six hours.

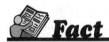 *Fact*

Some parents believe that if their child's temperature does not go down to normal after a fever reducer is given, whatever is causing the fever must be very serious. This is definitely untrue. Fever reducers do not reset the body temperature to normal. They only lower the temperature by a few degrees for a few hours.

A common misconception about fever reducers is that they make the fever go away. These medications, including acetaminophen and ibuprofen, do not work this way. Fever reducers simply lower the body temperature by a few degrees for a few hours. They do not necessarily return the body temperature to a normal level. They also cause parents to have unrealistic expectations, which can add to a parent's frustration and anxiety.

If your child's temperature does not decrease significantly with the fever reducer, it does not mean that she is more likely to have a bacterial than a viral infection. In addition, it does not mean that the cause of the fever is more critical either.

Medication Safety

It is commonly believed that since these medications are sold over the counter, they must be extraordinarily safe. But this is not entirely true. Even though they are harmless when taken at the recommended dose, administration of a higher dose or with greater frequency than instructed on the label can be detrimental to anyone's health. Many parents give repeated doses to their children because the initial dose fails to lower the fever back to normal, and some of them unintentionally overdose their children with Tylenol or Motrin.

Tylenol must not be given more often than every four hours, and Motrin must not be given more often than every six hours. It is essential not to confuse these instructions, which are clearly labeled on any medication bottle sold over the counter. In addition, consider the weight of your child when administering these medications. It is a more accurate way to calculate the dosage than by age alone. Simply follow the weight-based dosing table included with any fever reducer sold over the counter.

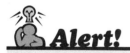

Alert!

Even though most parents already know that aspirin should not be given to children, it needs to be reiterated here. One of the most unfortunate misnomers ever given to a medication is "baby aspirin." The descriptor "baby" is used to refer to the small dose of the medication, not that this medication is meant for babies.

Tylenol overdose is not a benign condition. In fact, if it is not treated promptly, it leads to irreversible liver damage, which can be fatal and cause the need for a liver transplant. Unfortunately, most of the general public is not aware of the danger of Tylenol overdose. Excessive dosing of Tylenol is almost a daily occurrence during the flu season.

In addition, don't keep your child on fever reducers for more than four days without first seeking medical advice from a physician. If a fever lasts for more than four days, a serious underlying condition might be causing it. If you continue to lower the temperature after a few days, you are just masking whatever it is that might be triggering the fever. This could delay treatments. Bring your child to the doctor if the fever persists for more than four days.

CHAPTER 6

The Common Cold

Coughs and colds are by far the most common complaints pediatricians encounter. Most colds resolve spontaneously without serious consequences, but they can still be some of the most frustrating illnesses to treat. By arming yourself with more knowledge about the topic and having realistic expectations, you can better cope with the stresses and possibly see the light at the end of the tunnel as your child gets better.

Colds and the Weather

Even though most children with a cold get better in a few days, the severe cough and congestion that accompany a bad cold can make parents pretty desperate. You would do anything to make your sick child feel better. Unfortunately, there are a lot of misconceptions about the treatment for this common illness, and many therapies are misused. In addition, there are innumerable myths about how you can catch a cold.

The common belief that cold or changing weather causes illness is perhaps the mother of all myths. Not only is this cross-cultural, it's cross-generational as well. Even well-educated parents buy into this myth. Virtually everyone believes that you can get a cold by being exposed to cold weather or fluctuating temperatures.

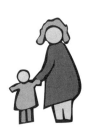

This association between cold weather and catching colds has more to do with seasonal human behavior. During the winter, people tend to gather in indoor environments more than they do during the warmer months. As people crowd together in close proximity, they are more likely to spread infections to one another. This hypothesis has not been substantiated by any rigor of science, but it does make intuitive sense.

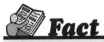

Fact

There is a real condition called vasomotor rhinitis. It happens in people who have very sensitive noses, so when their noses are exposed to cold air, they sneeze and get a runny nose. The symptoms can be very similar to having a cold, but they are temporary.

The True Cause of Colds

As you probably know already, a cold is a type of infection caused by a virus. There are over 200 different types of viruses that can cause the common cold, so over the course of your life you are bound to get sick on a regular basis, especially when there is a cold virus outbreak in the community. Even though it may seem like your doctor never gets sick, pediatricians probably get sick more often than other medical specialists.

Many parents go out of their way to reduce the likelihood of their children catching a cold. Blow-drying the hair immediately after a bath, taking a shower in the late afternoon instead of the morning, or wearing a jacket even in temperate weather are all practices people have tried to prevent colds. Unfortunately, none of these measures is beneficial in illness prevention.

The fact is that it is simply impossible to get sick from not dressing adequately or going out with wet hair. You will only get a cold if you're exposed to a virus.

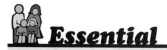

Essential

It's impossible to "pass around" a cold back and forth between family members. Once someone gets sick from one type of virus, her body becomes immune to that specific virus for a long while. Nevertheless, it's still possible to get a cold again right after getting sick because there are just so many types of viruses out there to make you sick.

Even though people don't get sick purely from cold exposure, having a lower temperature in the nose may make someone more likely to get sick if he or she is already exposed to the virus. Recent studies show that if the temperature in the nose is lowered, a person is less able than a person with a warm nose to fight off an invading cold virus. A simple exposure to cold still won't make you sick, but if you're exposed to a virus at the same time, you are more likely to come down with a cold. This may be caused by the fact that immune cells don't work as well when the body's temperature is lower, making them less effective in warding off a viral invasion.

Notorious Green Mucus

The fear of green mucus is so deeply entrenched that even some health-care professionals still incorrectly believe it. Thousands of parents bring their children to the doctor's office unnecessarily each year because they fear that green mucus means that their child has come down with a bacterial infection.

Green mucus does not necessarily indicate the presence of a bacterial infection. In fact, when nasal discharge turns green, it usually means that whatever is causing the mucus in the first place is retreating. As a person recovers from a cold, the amount of nasal discharge decreases, and the mucus naturally thickens. This often changes the color of the mucus from clear to yellow or green. The underlying reasons for nasal discharge are many, including a viral infection, nasal allergy, some object that got stuck inside the nostril, or a bacterial infection of the sinuses. The fact that the secretion is green doesn't provide any information about what might be causing the discharge.

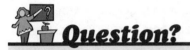

Question?

What causes the mucus to turn green?
The green color has nothing to do with the presence of bacteria. In fact, the green color appears because one of the chemicals produced by the body's own immune cells appears green. This type of immune cell can appear in many scenarios, including infections and allergy.

The only situation in which mucus discharge makes it necessary to use antibiotics is when there is a bacterial infection, most frequently caused by an infection in the sinus. However, this typically occurs after at least two weeks of runny nose and nasal congestion. Other symptoms, including body aches, headache, or low-grade fever may also help the diagnosis of a sinus infection. A true sinus infection is almost never the problem when the green mucus has been around for just a few days.

Milk and Mucus

Most people believe that when they are sick with a cough, they should avoid milk or dairy products in general because this type of food will generate more phlegm and make their cough worse. This is an extremely popular misconception, and it's cross-generational as well as cross-cultural.

This myth may have arisen from the sensation many people feel after they drink milk. It's a sticky sensation at the back of the throat, as though something was coating it. An Australian hospital has conducted a study in which they had fifty-one healthy volunteers willingly infect themselves with a cold virus, and the researchers measured the amount of snot they subsequently produced. The consumption of milk varied from eleven glasses a day to none at all, but the "snot production" factor had no correlation with the amount of milk they drank. Scientists have sought to discredit the belief of increased phlegm production because this myth has actually reduced the consumption of dairy products in the past.

In fact, milk might even improve cold symptoms because it is a good source of fluid and nutrition. It's jam-packed with vitamins and protein, providing the body with fuel and raw material for building more germ-fighting cells. So drink up! Milk really does a body good, even when you're sick.

Of course, if your child is already feeling nauseated and threw up the last time she tried drinking milk, don't force the issue. It's not that the milk will make more mucus, but if your child can't keep the milk down, there is no point in trying to drink and throwing up right afterward.

Cold Remedies for Infants

For treating children less than two years old (some experts say three years), there simply isn't any medication that can relieve cold symptoms. In fact, pediatricians know this from an established body of research involving hundreds of children who have been treated with cold medicines—decongestants and cough suppressants. For children less than three years, there is no proven benefit from these medications. Most of them would probably be better off if parents blew kisses at them because at least the kisses would not cause any side effects.

While it is true that most of these medications are quite safe in older children, the risk for infants is often overlooked by parents and even health professionals. If given appropriately at the right dose and interval, there would be no harm done in most cases. But why should you give something to your child that doesn't help at all and risk even the small possibility of adverse reactions?

 Essential

If you take a close look at any cold remedy designed for young children, you will find that they do not provide any dosage information for children under the age of two. Instead, they recommend the buyer to "consult your doctor." What the label really should say is "This medication does not work for children under two, so please do not buy it."

The Antibiotic Myth

Many parents believe that antibiotics are the only thing that can make a sick child better. Even though parents are usually quite satisfied after the pediatrician has given them a detailed explanation of their child's condition, there are plenty of situations when a visit to the doctor can become a source of frustration and dismay. If parents clamor for a prescription of antibiotics when doctors recommend against it, the encounter can become tense. At the end of such a visit, both the parents and the doctor are worn out.

This type of confrontation clearly isn't necessary. Parents and doctor are both acting in the best interest of the child, so there really shouldn't be any conflict of interest. There is no reason why any doctor would withhold the appropriate treatment when it is indicated. If parents understand the reason behind the doctor's reluctance in handing out antibiotics, the doctor-patient relationship can be significantly improved.

A Case of Misunderstanding

In fact, this parental pressure for pediatricians to prescribe antibiotics is so overwhelming that many pediatricians go out of their way to avoid using the word "infection" with parents. The second this word is uttered, parents tend to set their minds on getting a prescription for antibiotics for their child's illness, and the remainder of the visit becomes a battle of the wills between the doctor and the parents.

Some parents find it unreasonable and incredible that the doctor would withhold an essential form of treatment from their child. As far as they are concerned, the doctor isn't doing the right thing. Not giving an antibiotic prescription means that the doctor simply doesn't care.

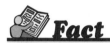

Fact

Antibiotics are completely useless against infections caused by viruses, whereas they are sometimes useful against bacteria. Doctors do not use antibiotics against viruses because it does not make any sense to pre-scribe a medication that is completely ineffective in the given situation.

Types of Infections

Ultimately, infections can be caused by a wide range of organisms, including viruses, bacteria, fungi, and parasites. Aside from the more exotic causes and origins, the vast majority of childhood infections are caused by viruses and bacteria. It is crucial to understand this distinction because the approach to treatment is entirely different.

Antibiotics can frequently shorten the duration of a bacterial infection. In some cases, antibiotic use plays an essential role in the cure of and recovery from the infection. At the same time, antibiotics are not always able to help treat all bacterial infections. Your doctor is well trained in deciding whether it is necessary to use antibiotics to fight an infection.

Bacterial meningitis is an example of an illness caused by bacterial infection. It is a very serious and potentially fatal infection of the tissues covering the brain. No doctor would hesitate in treating bacterial meningitis with antibiotics. Other common childhood bacterial infections include pneumonia, bone and joint infections, and skin infections.

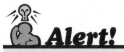
Alert!

Not all bacterial infections should be treated with antibiotics. In some cases, managing certain types of bacterial infections with antibiotics can actually make things worse. For example, when a patient with typhoid fever is treated with antibiotics, the treatment prolongs the infection instead of treating it.

On the other hand, ear infections (covered in more detail in Chapter 7) may or may not need to be treated with antibiotics. European health providers have successfully been using an observational approach (that is, not prescribing antibiotics for all ear infections) when managing ear infections. Viruses cause a significant percentage of ear infections, and even those caused by bacteria frequently resolve without medical intervention.

CHAPTER 7

Ear Infections

The majority of children will get a few ear infections during childhood, and it is a common enough pediatric issue to deserve its own chapter. Although most ear infections resolve uneventfully, there are some potentially serious consequences that might complicate an ear infection. In addition, the management of ear infections is not always as straightforward as you might expect. Controversies, even within the professional medical community, can make it tricky for a parent trying to do the right thing for a child.

Introducing the Ear

Most people are very familiar with their external ears because they are visible and easily accessible. However, the internal structures of ears and the associated hearing apparatus are much more obscure. The external ear only acts as a physical siphon for sounds. It funnels the sound waves and allows the vibration to be passed into the eardrum, where its vibration is subsequently transformed into nerve signals that can be interpreted by the brain. What makes hearing possible is this intricate system of tubes and ducts, some of which are hollow and some that are filled with fluid. The presence of infection disrupts this delicate mechanism. Ultimately, what pediatricians

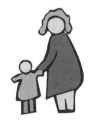

and parents are most concerned about is preserving normal functionality of hearing.

Ear Anatomy

The anatomy of the ear is divided into three major sections. The external ear is the part of the ear that you can see, extending all the way to the eardrum. The middle ear resides between the eardrum and the inner ear, where the nerves responsible for hearing are located. The middle ear is mostly filled with air, whereas the inner ear is mostly filled with fluid.

The inner structure of the ear is truly a work of wonder. Along with the small tubes that are designed to transmit sound waves, there is a complex drainage system network that allows certain internal structures of the ear to be filled with air and at a pressure equal to the outside environment. Without such a system, the hearing apparatus could not function properly.

In order to maintain this equal pressure, the internal air pocket is connected to the throat via a small duct. This duct is called the Eustachian tube.

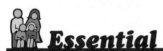 **Essential**

Given that the external ear and the middle ear are separated by a physical barrier (the eardrum), it is virtually impossible to get a middle ear infection from swimming. Swimmers can get swimmer's ear, which is an infection of the external ear. This has nothing to do with the typical ear infection, which is an infection of the middle ear.

The Eustachian tube is very small, and it can open and close its connection to the throat at will. Most of the time, the duct is sealed off to prevent food and mucus from entering the air pocket inside the ear. It opens briefly when you open your jaw, swallow, or yawn.

Individual Differences

Just as all people have unique facial features, the internal structure of the ear is also quite varied. The shape of the Eustachian tube that equalizes the pressure inside the ear is different in everyone. Some people have long and narrow tubes, while others have thick and short ones. Depending on the configuration of the tube, some tubes are more likely to stay open than others. The long and narrow ones tend to get clogged with mucus more easily.

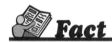 **Fact**

During air travel, the cabin pressure of the airplane is somewhat lower than the atmospheric pressure at sea level. Consequently, the Eustachian tube must open briefly to balance the pressure difference inside the middle ear and the cabin. It is a good idea to give your infant something to drink during these times because she cannot voluntarily yawn or swallow to open up her Eustachian tube.

If the tube becomes obstructed, fluid tends to accumulate inside the middle ear, an area normally filled with air. Once this fluid settles into the middle ear, the risk of infection goes way up. The fact that some people's Eustachian tubes are more easily blocked than others is the reason why some children tend to suffer from more frequent ear infections. In addition, children tend to have smaller tubes, a configuration that makes them more likely to get clogged with mucus when they have a cold. That is the reason why children get ear infections more often than adults.

The Origin of Ear Infection

As explained earlier, the Eustachian tube plays a crucial role in regulating the pressure inside the middle ear. Once the tube stops working, the abnormal pressure inside the middle ear causes fluid to accumulate there. This stagnant fluid, which is rich in protein and sugar, is an ideal growth medium for bacteria. If the pressure does not normalize quickly, bacteria flourish in this fluid, starting an infection in the middle ear. When doctors use the term "ear infection," they are generally referring to a middle ear infection.

In short, whenever the Eustachian tube does not function normally, the chance of getting an ear infection increases. There are several situations in which the functionality of the Eustachian tube may be impaired.

The Common Cold

Among all the possible risk factors for triggering an ear infection, catching a cold is by far the most common. When your child has a cold, his nose and throat are usually stuffed with mucus. Since the Eustachian tube connects the middle ear and the throat, it is easy for the excessive secretion to compromise the function of the tube. Once the Eustachian tube is blocked, it may be just a matter of time before your child comes down with an ear infection, especially if he is prone to getting them.

Consequently, the best way to prevent an ear infection is to avoid catching a cold. The most effective strategy for avoiding a cold is frequent hand washing.

Nasal Allergy

Someone with chronic and recurrent ear infections also often suffers from nasal allergy. Similar to having a cold, a child with nasal allergy has constant excessive secretion in the nose and throat. This abundance of mucus blocks the Eustachian tube and increases the child's chance of getting an ear infection.

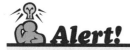
Alert!

If your child suffers from frequent ear infections, it is very important to make sure that she does not have untreated nasal allergy. Treating each episode of ear infection will only make the symptoms go away temporarily. It may not solve the nasal allergy that is the culprit for triggering all the infections.

Unfortunately, these children frequently return to the doctor's office for ear infections over and over again, and they take antibiotics repeatedly for these episodes. In some cases they are never treated for the real cause of these recurrent ear infections. It is important to remember that as long as a child's nasal allergy is not controlled, she is at high risk for getting more ear infections. The most important thing is for the doctors treating these children to recognize the presence of their allergy and treat the allergy with appropriate medication. Otherwise, the children are doomed to suffer this terrible problem of constant ear pain. Some of them might even receive surgery unnecessarily because of their multiple infections. (The role of surgery in treating ear infection is addressed on page 87).

Unusual Anatomy

Differences in the shape and configuration of the Eustachian tube can cause some children to suffer from ear infections more frequently than others, as stated previously. Other anatomical structures, including the size and position of the tongue and the overall shape of the head, can also indirectly influence the functionality of the Eustachian tube.

For example, children with Down syndrome tend to have larger tongues, which is more likely to obstruct the opening of the Eustachian tube. Children with smaller heads as a result of other medical conditions have more ear infections because their tubes are smaller as well. The bottom line is that a working Eustachian tube is paramount in preventing ear infections.

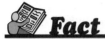 **Fact**

Excessive earwax is frequently blamed for causing ear infections. This is completely untrue. In fact, earwax is quite acidic, and the presence of earwax in the external ear canals tends to prevent the development of swimmer's ear (external ear infection). The presence of earwax has nothing to do with middle ear infection, other than making it difficult for doctors to evaluate the eardrums.

Signs of Infection

One of the widely believed myths in pediatrics is that if your child pulls his ears, then he must have an ear infection. Even though this can be true in some circumstances, this behavior is a red herring in many cases. There are many symptoms associated with ear infections, and pulling on the ears is one of the least reliable. This section describes the various ways you can recognize an ear infection in your child. The presence of any single one of these symptoms may not be very helpful in determining the likelihood of ear infection. They must be considered together to assemble the whole picture.

Things That May Indicate an Infection

There are many factors that increase a pediatrician's suspicion that ear infection may be present, including the following.

Runny Nose

A runny nose is one of the symptoms most likely to occur along with an ear infection. In fact, a middle ear infection is unlikely to occur without some increased nasal secretion. If your child has a stuffy or runny nose for a few days, then suddenly starts to develop other symptoms of ear infection, it is quite possible that he has come down with an infection in the ear.

Crankiness

Crankiness is a very generic response from an ill child. He may be cranky for a lot of reasons, but ear infection must be one of the considerations. Simply having a cold often makes a child irritable, but the degree of irritability may be higher from the intense pain that originates from an ear infection. Parents are astonishingly good at recognizing an increase in the level of distress in their children, and pediatricians must heed their instinct.

Fever

Not all ear infections trigger a fever, and not all fever indicates the presence of an ear infection. Fever is a very nonspecific finding, but it may be a helpful clue in determining the presence of an ear infection. Like all other symptoms described in this section, it must be considered as one of the pieces of the puzzle.

Drainage from the Ear

If liquid, either white or pus-like, drains out from the ear, it usually means your child has an ear infection. While this might indicate a middle ear infection serious enough that it has caused the eardrum to rupture, it could also suggest the presence of the infection known as swimmer's ear, which only involves the external ear. Whether your child has a middle or external ear infection can be determined only by a health professional.

Vomiting and Diarrhea

Ear infections can also cause some seemingly unrelated problems, such as nausea, cough, vomiting, or diarrhea. When the ears are inflamed, the infection may irritate the throat and trigger a cough reflex. In addition, the nerve that controls equilibrium traverses through the middle ear. An infection of the middle ear could aggravate this nerve and cause dizziness, upsetting the stomach.

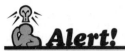

Alert!

The external ear canals should never be cleaned with cotton swabs like Q-tips. Cotton swabs are designed for removing makeup and cleaning computer keyboards. They have no place inside your child's ears. Using cotton swabs to clean the ears risks perforating the eardrum and causing permanent damage to the ears.

Ear-Infection Mimics

When diagnosing ear infections, most pediatricians inquire about additional symptoms that make ear infection less likely. Many confounding factors can make a child appear to have ear pain when in fact she does not.

Of course, it is important to keep the age of the child in mind. Beyond a certain age, usually between three or four years, most children can reliably report ear pain when it is present. It may take quite a bit of guesswork to ascertain whether younger children are experiencing discomfort in their ears.

Teething

Teething causes an uncomfortable sensation in the gums. Infants cannot verbalize their discomfort and they cannot accurately localize the source of their pain. Frequently, when infants are teething, they bat on the side of their heads or ears because they sense the discomfort of teething. Parents commonly misinterpret this gesture as a sign of ear pain.

Exploration of the Body

Many infants less than a year old love to use their fingers to explore the various parts of their bodies. Having just mastered rudimentary control of their hands, they enjoy touching their toes, faces, and ears. The external ear is interestingly shaped, and its novel form is fascinating to many children. Having an ear on either side of their heads is almost like having two toys that are attached there. The ears are very convenient to play with because they will never drop to the ground.

This type of exploration is most common between the ages of nine and fifteen months. Beyond that age, children typically do not play with their ears without a reason.

Eustachian Tube Dysfunction

When the Eustachian tube is blocked by mucus, hearing can be partially impaired because the pressure difference between the air pocket in the middle ear and the outside environment increases. Older children often describe this as "muffled" hearing. Even though this condition is not the same as having an ear infection, it can be a precursor of an ear infection. If your child describes this type of sensation, have her checked by the doctor to confirm the presence or absence of infection in the ear.

Headache

Babies do get headaches. When they do, they have no way of expressing their annoyance. Many of them end up hitting the side of their head, which can make their parents believe that they are experiencing pain in the ears. This is just another situation in which ear poking or pulling does not necessarily indicate the presence of ear infection.

Prevention Is the Key

Now that you understand what causes ear infections, you naturally want to know how to prevent them. As stated previously, hand washing is one of the best ways to prevent ear infections because it reduces your child's chance of getting a cold in the first place. Controlling nasal allergy with medication and other avoidance measures is another way to thwart the onset of ear infections. However, there are additional factors that can be managed to further reduce the risk of getting an ear infection.

Day Care

Simply being in a day-care setting increases the likelihood that your child will have frequent bouts of viral illnesses. Children do not tend to have the best hygiene practices. When they play together, they share the same toys and frequently touch each other. Furthermore, a child's immune system is more immature than that of an adult because the child has not been exposed to as many infections over the years as the adult. All these factors contribute to the perfect setting for the transmission of germs.

As you have learned, nasal congestion is almost a prerequisite for the development of an ear infection. If children catch more colds in the day-care environment, they are also a lot more likely to have frequent ear infections. Unfortunately, it is not always possible to simply take your children out of day care. It is possible, however, to ensure that your child's day-care facility has good standards of hygiene and that it makes it a practice to have as few children as possible in the same area. Beyond these considerations, the situation is usually out of your control.

Bottle to the Bed

As children grow up, it is often difficult for them to give up the last bottle of the day, one that they might be accustomed to taking to bed. An older child might be able to make it through the entire day without needing a bottle, but at the end of the day, she feels comforted by the nighttime bottle. It's part of her bedtime routine.

In addition to the increased risk of developing cavities, letting a child have a bedtime bottle has another negative side effect. It increases the chance of developing ear infections. It is believed that the milk consumed while the child is lying on his back could backflow from his throat via the Eustachian tube into the middle ear cavity. This style of feeding could fill the middle ear with a small amount of residual milk, thereby encouraging bacteria overgrowth inside the ear.

 Essential

It may be extremely difficult to cajole your child into quitting his night-time bottle cold turkey. Instead, you can give him water to drink or have him drink his bottle sitting up instead of lying down. Make sure that he cleans his teeth after the bottle is finished and before he goes to sleep. This will help prevent cavities.

Secondhand Smoke

Secondhand smoke kills. It is a medical fact that has been proven beyond any doubt over the past years. Nevertheless, it is still a fact of life in many households. Not only can it cause cancers of the throat and lungs in the long run, it can also exacerbate asthma and worsen allergy symptoms. It has been clearly shown that microscopic smoke particles impair clearing of secretions in the throat because the toxins in these particles paralyze the mucus-clearing mechanism of the throat and the lungs. Once this mechanism is botched, secretion in the throat increases, and the excessive mucus blocks the Eustachian tube and causes ear infections.

The Role of Antibiotics

It used to be a simple matter for the pediatrician when an ear infection was diagnosed. Antibiotics were routinely prescribed to stave off the infection and relieve symptoms. However, new findings from recent medical research have complicated the process by suggesting it may be better to treat the patient symptomatically instead of using antibiotics in all cases. This is one of the most controversial topics in pediatrics today. It seems every doctor has a different approach to the treatment of ear infections.

The European Standard

More and more doctors are managing ear infections with careful observation and close follow-ups, especially if the child is older and the symptoms are mild. Though physicians in Europe have been doing this for decades, this style of treatment has only started making its way into the United States in the past few years. In fact, the American Academy of Pediatrics has recently incorporated this recommendation into its official guidelines.

This conservative approach in managing ear infections has many advantages. First of all, the majority of ear infections get better without medical treatment. Some research demonstrates that as many as 80 percent of all ear infections get better in less than a week without the use of antibiotics. There are many reasons why this happens. Healthy children have an intact immune system, which is more than adequate to conquer most ear infections. In the vast majority of cases, the immune system is able to quell an ear infection before antibiotics even have the chance to kick in.

Secondly, it is viruses rather than bacteria that are responsible for causing more than half of all ear infections. In the case of a viral ear infection, using antibiotics would not make the patient feel any better or recover any faster. Antibiotics are only capable of treating infections caused by bacteria. They are completely useless against viruses. This is another reason doctors do not immediately get out the prescription pad for every ear infection.

Vaccine for Ear Infection

It is a common but mistaken belief that scientists have developed a vaccine to curtail ear infections. This myth originated from the introduction in 2000 of a new vaccine against a bacterium called pneumococcus. This vaccine carries the trade name Prevnar, and the bacteria that it is designed to fight is the most common cause of ear infections. Many people concluded that if the vaccine was effective against this bacterium, then it must be able to reduce the cases of ear infections.

Unfortunately, it's not that simple. Even though pneumococcus causes more ear infections than any other bacteria, there are still many other bacteria that trigger ear infections. In addition, there are more than ten different strains of the pneumococcus bacterium that can cause serious illnesses. The Prevnar vaccine only protects against seven of these strains. Finally, this vaccine obviously does not prevent ear infections that are caused by viruses.

If this vaccine is no good for ear infections, why was it developed? It turns out that these few strains of pneumococcal bacteria cause the majority of cases of pneumonia and meningitis (brain infection) in young children. The incentive to curb these serious infections was the impetus for the creation of this vaccine. It was never intended to prevent ear infections. Consequently, while pediatricians still recommend this highly effective and useful vaccine, it is a mistake to believe that this series of shots will protect your child from getting any ear infections in the future.

The Role of Surgery

While surgery definitely has a role in the management of recurrent ear infections, it does not guarantee that a child will be completely free of ear infections in the future. Other factors need to be considered prior to resorting to a surgical solution.

Ear Tubes

How does surgery help to curb recurrent ear infections? The premise of the surgery is rather straightforward. As you already understand, ear infections occur when the Eustachian tube fails to drain the fluid from the middle ear. Since surgeons cannot remodel the internal structure of the Eustachian tube easily, they add an alternative route for drainage of the fluid. Instead of having the middle ear fluid drain through the Eustachian tube and into the throat, surgeons create a small hole in the eardrum and place a small plastic tube through the aperture to keep it open. Without this plastic tube, the eardrum would quickly heal itself and seal up the hole within a week or two.

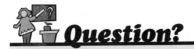 **Question?**

When should ear-tube surgery be considered for a child suffering from ear infections?
Most pediatricians start to think about the possibility of ear-tube placement if a child has suffered from more than five ear infections within a twelve-month period. In addition, an ear infection that fails to resolve after three months of antibiotic treatment should prompt most doctors to at least consider surgery.

The technical aspect of this surgery is relatively easy. Most surgeons can adeptly accomplish it within half an hour. However, the downside of this procedure does not lie in the surgery itself. The greatest risk for a child undergoing this intervention is the anesthesia involved. In order to perform the surgery with the child completely motionless, surgeons need to sedate the child completely, using general anesthesia. This means that your child must be put to sleep and completely paralyzed during the procedure. Even though most children do well under anesthesia, a small percentage experience serious reactions. While the exact level of risk is difficult to generalize for all pediatric patients, this is a risk for any child undergoing elective surgery.

The Overlooked Allergy

It is not uncommon for children suffering from nasal allergy to be referred for ear-tube placement when their allergy symptoms have not been controlled. For these children, the ear tubes often fail to provide relief. This is because the underlying reason for their numerous ear infections has not been properly dealt with.

Instead of immediately being subjected to the surgical option, children with frequent ear infections need to first be evaluated for nasal allergy. More often than not, after their nasal allergy is under control, they experience a dramatic reduction in ear infection frequency. Most of these children will never require surgery to cure their problem with chronic ear infections.

The bottom line is that ear-tube placement should be considered the treatment of last resort for ear infections. Other means of reducing ear infections, such as taking a low-dose antibiotic on a daily basis, could be considered prior to opting for surgery.

A Temporary Solution

Before having your children undergo ear-tube surgery, you must understand that the placement of ear tubes may offer only a temporary respite from infections. Once these tubes are placed through the eardrums, they are destined to fall out sooner or later, usually within nine to eighteen months. In some unfortunate patients, these tubes are rejected by the body in less than six months. Having the tubes stay in the eardrums is completely harmless. They do not affect your child's hearing. However, there is no way to predict how long the tubes are going to stay in place once they are inserted.

It's not uncommon for some children to have this surgery repeatedly because the tubes fall out so quickly. Frequent surgeries increase the chance of anesthesia complication for these children, which is another reason parents should hesitate before submitting their children to surgery over and over again.

CHAPTER 8

Digestive Troubles

Vomiting and diarrhea are the banes of the pediatrician's existence. Perhaps due to the prevalence of stomach problems, there is a wealth of old wives' tales and remedies about vomiting and diarrhea. Surprisingly, most of the alleged age-old wisdom is not helpful in these situations, and it can even be harmful. Before you venture out and follow your great-aunt's advice for curing your child's diarrhea, make sure you have the facts straight.

Baby Spit-Ups

Acid reflux disease plagues many adults. While reflux can also occur in babies, baby reflux is not the same as adult reflux. For one thing, unlike the adult form of the condition, reflux in babies does not increase the risk of ulcer or cancer. In addition, reflux is far more common in otherwise healthy babies than it is in adults. Most importantly, infantile reflux is mostly a benign condition, and affected babies almost always grow out of their reflux condition in a matter of months.

Anatomy Lesson
To understand reflux and other intestinal conditions, it is necessary that you first become acquainted with some basic anatomy. Let's follow the path of the food your baby eats after he swallows it.

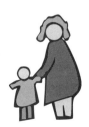

The esophagus is a long and narrow tube made of muscle that connects the mouth to the stomach. Before the food makes it to the esophagus, it must stay clear of the windpipe first. Any food that goes into the wrong tube could have disastrous consequences. For this reason, all babies are equipped right at birth with a sophisticated muscle-control system that prevents this from happening.

Every time your baby swallows, an automatic trap door covers up the entrance to the windpipe to prevent food from going down the wrong pipe. This system of control is so essential that it is intact even in many brain-damaged babies. It is absent only in the most severely neurologically impaired children.

 Essential

If your baby has reflux, your pediatrician may want to measure the baby's weight frequently to ensure that he is thriving. Your baby's weight gain is the most important indicator that everything is going well and that no medical intervention is necessary for his reflux.

When the food reaches the stomach, a muscular gateway briefly opens up to allow the food to enter the stomach. This valve technically only allows food to go from the esophagus into the stomach. As you'll learn later, this valve doesn't always work perfectly.

Once the food is inside the stomach, it gets churned around for a while, and some of the water in the food passes through the stomach lining and into the body. Once the churning is complete, another one-way gateway opens up, and the food is transported into the intestine. Like a hyped-up bouncer, this second valve sometimes becomes overzealous, as we'll discuss later. Problems occur when it is hyperactive and doesn't allow food to pass through its door.

Reflux Management

Food is only supposed to move in one direction, from the esophagus to the stomach. Once the food is inside the stomach, it should not go back up into the esophagus or the mouth. In babies with reflux, however, this is not the case.

The stomach valve in these babies is not sealed very tightly. So as the stomach churns the food, the content sometimes spills out. Imagine a malfunctioning zip-close bag full of last night's clam chowder. If the bag isn't tightly sealed, and you start jiggling the bag violently, you're going to end up with a big mess in the kitchen.

Fortunately, as the baby grows older, the function of the valve steadily improves. By the time the baby is nine months to a year old, most babies with reflux should stop spitting up. Until the condition resolves, the most important thing is that these babies retain enough calories to gain weight. As long as your baby can take in enough calories to grow, it doesn't matter how much milk he's spitting up. It is messy and inconvenient, but spitting up in a thriving baby is entirely harmless.

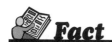 **Fact**

It is a good idea to keep your baby upright or at least inclined immediately after feeding. This way, gravity will help the food to settle into the stomach instead of being churned up and purged out. Avoid moving the baby excessively after feeding. In addition, burping the baby more often may reduce spit-ups.

Occasionally, some babies throw up so much that they stop growing. If this is the case with your child, your doctor will first prescribe a medication to control the vomiting and recommend you to thicken up the baby's milk with some rice cereal. If that fails to improve weight gain, a surgical procedure might be considered to tighten up the stomach muscle. Keep in mind that surgery is really the last resort, and most pediatricians will not consider it until all else has failed. The expertise of a pediatric gastroenterologist is often requested when persistent or difficult-to-control reflux is present.

Projectile Vomiting

Projectile vomiting is dangerous in babies. Not only are parents easy targets around such a baby, but this type of forceful vomiting could indicate something more serious about the baby's stomach. Doctors worry about this type of vomiting because it could be a sign of pyloric stenosis. Pyloric stenosis is when the baby's stomach muscle is too tight to allow food to pass through the stomach into the intestines.

This condition is potentially life threatening because it could cause the baby to become dehydrated and lose weight. Pyloric stenosis is more common in boys, but it can happen in either gender. It usually doesn't affect the baby right from birth, but develops slowly and finally rears its ugly head when the baby is three to six weeks old.

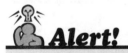

Alert!

All babies spit up in large quantities at one time or another. Sometimes the milk even comes out of their noses. If forceful vomiting is infrequent, there is usually no cause for concern. However, if you see that the frequency of vomiting is increasing and your baby is unable to keep milk down, call your pediatrician.

Babies who are affected with pyloric stenosis initially tolerate feeding just fine, but they start throwing up around four weeks old. This vomiting gradually increases in frequency and force until it eventually occurs after almost every feeding. The baby usually appears very hungry but cannot keep the milk down. The projectile strength is impressive. The spit-up is large in quantity and can literally shoot across the room and splatter against the wall. If your baby is doing this, contact your pediatrician immediately.

Pyloric stenosis can be easily cured with a relatively small surgical procedure that takes less than an hour for an experienced surgeon to complete. Your baby might not be able to feed immediately after the surgery, but recovery is typically rapid. Most babies leave the hospital after only a day or two.

Bloody Stools

It's understandably alarming to detect blood in your child's stool. Fortunately, this relatively common occurrence usually indicates a benign condition. If you believe you have found blood in your baby's diaper, it's very helpful if you can bring that diaper to the doctor's office to show it to your pediatrician directly. Wrap the diaper up and seal it in a zip-close bag. Schedule the earliest appointment you can so that the stool is still fresh when the doctor looks at it. Don't worry; pediatricians are used to seeing vomit and stools.

Fake Blood

A red hue in the stool doesn't always indicate the presence of blood. Frequently, a very convincing-looking bloody stool turns out to take its color from traces of tomato or colored fruit drinks instead. The doctor can perform a quick and easy chemical analysis to detect even minute traces of blood. If this test returns a negative result, the redness in the stool must be something other than blood.

This test cannot be performed unless you bring the stool in question to the doctor's office. A look really is worth a thousand words.

Anal Fissure

Anal fissure occurs when the stool stretches the skin a little too much around the anus, causing it to tear. This is perhaps the most common reason for actual blood to appear in the stool of infants and older children. The child may or may not complain of pain during defecation, as the tear may be so tiny that it doesn't really hurt. A history of constipation or hard stool is common but not mandatory for this condition to occur.

If the blood in the stool is caused by anal fissure, the blood is usually just on the surface of the stool. Sometimes it is difficult to tell whether the blood is just on the surface or mixed in with the stool, especially if the stool is not well formed. If the stool is hard enough, you can frequently see a linear streak of redness on the surface of the stool as it comes out of the anus.

Surprisingly, anal fissures tend to heal themselves fairly quickly. Even in this area of constant bacterial contamination, infection is rare. Make sure your child's stools stay soft, and the absence of hard stools will usually allow the anal fissure to heal itself. Application of creams or ointment is not necessary.

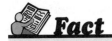 **Fact**

The pediatrician needs to examine the anus directly, perhaps even with a magnifying scope, to evaluate the presence of anal fissure. Don't worry; doctors usually do not have to stick a finger into the anus to find a fissure.

Milk Protein Allergy

Allergy to cow's-milk protein is a fairly common problem in babies. If your baby spits up excessively and has traces of blood mixed in her stool, she might be allergic to cow's milk. This could occur if you are feeding your baby commercial infant formula or are breastfeeding and taking in a significant amount of dairy product.

The first step in diagnosing cow's-milk protein allergy is to make a trip to your doctor's. The pediatrician will make sure that there is actual blood in the stools and that the bloody stools aren't caused by something else (such as an anal fissure). When milk protein allergy is suspected, your child's doctor will usually recommend an alternative soy-based formula or, if you are breastfeeding, may ask you to restrict dairy products from your diet. If the throwing up stops and the stool normalizes, the problem is solved.

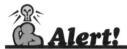

Alert!

Many children who are allergic to cow's-milk protein are also allergic to soy protein. If the symptoms of cow's-milk allergy do not resolve after switching to a soy-based food source, it's possible that your child may also be allergic to soy. Talk to your doctor if this happens.

Fortunately, most infants grow out of their milk allergies as they get older. Exactly when this happens is anyone's guess, but it's not unreasonable to test again for cow's-milk protein allergy when your child is four or five years old.

The Stomach Virus

Many people refer to infections that are caused by a stomach virus as the stomach flu. This is a highly misleading term because this type of stomach infection has absolutely nothing to do with the flu virus that occurs every winter. These viruses are completely unrelated, and the illnesses they cause have nothing in common.

Dirty Hands

The most common way to catch a stomach virus is from contaminated hands. If your child touches an object or another child's skin that is contaminated with the virus, the virus immediately transfers to your child's hand. After this initial step, it's just a matter of time before your child sticks his dirty hand inside his mouth. This is how a stomach virus gains entrance into the body.

Given that children between the age of six months and three years love putting everything inside their mouths, this is the age group most likely to be affected by these viral infections. The only ways to prevent the virus is to practice frequent hand washing and to avoid other sick children.

Stomach Virus Versus Food Poisoning

While most children get sick because of their frequent hand-to-mouth contact, eating contaminated foods is the more common way for adults to contract stomach viruses. Food poisoning differs from stomach virus in that food poisoning is caused by a bacterial toxin instead of a virus. A true case of food poisoning is not contagious, and vomiting tends to be more severe but shorter in duration than with infection from stomach viruses. It may take up to a few days after catching a virus before someone starts showing symptoms, whereas food poisoning can trigger bouts of vomiting within a few hours after the contaminated food is consumed.

Most food poisoning problems last less than twelve hours, but an attack from a stomach virus can last many days. The younger the victim, the longer the diarrhea lasts for a stomach viral infection.

Signs of Dehydration

The most important thing to prevent during a bout of intestinal problems is dehydration. Babies are more susceptible to becoming dehydrated than older children. This is because they have less of a water reservoir in their bodies to begin with due to their overall small size. Infants can become moderately dehydrated after even a few hours of not drinking. Toddlers are a lot more resistant to dehydration. Typically, they can go for a day or two without significant fluid intake before they succumb to dehydration.

 Essential

In babies, a sure sign of dehydration is if the soft spot on your baby's head appears to be sunken. However, this is a very late finding. By the time your baby's soft spot is sunken, your baby is already severely dehydrated and needs immediate medical intervention to reverse the condition. Look for early signs of dehydration, and do not rely on the soft spot to alert you to the gravity of the situation.

In order to detect dehydration, it's important that parents know what to look for. The first thing that changes when your child becomes dehydrated is her activity level. A dehydrated child becomes listless and tired when there isn't enough water in the body to keep her brain functioning at an optimal level. Some children become sleepy, while others become cranky. A baby might sleep longer and be difficult to wake up at feeding time. Even though these findings are not specific to dehydration, meaning they can also be signs of other conditions, you should consult your doctor when you observe these symptoms in your child.

Another useful physical finding in evaluating dehydration is the amount of moisture in your child's mouth. If you swipe your finger inside your child's mouth and it comes out wet, chances are your child is reasonably hydrated. If your finger is dry, you should call your pediatrician to schedule a visit.

Finally, you can tell whether your child is dehydrated by the amount of urine she's producing. This may be a tough finding to confirm, especially in babies. Today's diapers are so super-absorbent that it can be hard to ascertain how much urine they have soaked up. Older children may also use the bathroom without telling you, and they might forget how many times they have emptied their bladders. If you are concerned, you can monitor your infant's urine production more closely by putting a sheet of tissue paper inside her diaper. You can also monitor the frequency of your older child's bathroom visits.

Even though urine production is more difficult to monitor, it is a more reliable sign than other indicators. Your pediatrician may even ask you whether you have been checking urine production when you bring your child to the office. If it is feasible, recording such information could be a tremendous help to the doctor in making medical decisions.

Managing Diarrhea

Fortunately, most cases of intestinal problems aren't serious, and the vast majority of them resolve without any medical intervention. The culprit in most cases is viral, meaning that the infection will get better without any antibiotics. This also means that doing additional blood or stool laboratory tests is not only unnecessary but impractical. Plus, not many parents look for the opportunity to collect their toddler's stool sample and send it to the laboratory for analysis.

Treating a toddler who has the runs can be extremely frustrating. You have to make sure that your child is drinking enough fluid to prevent getting dehydrated. And you cannot use any antidiarrheal medication for your child.

The best fluid to offer your child initially is water. If she is unable to keep water down, she will not be able to drink anything else. It is essential to offer the fluid slowly, perhaps one teaspoon at a time. You cannot allow your child to gulp the fluid down, even if she is very thirsty. Doing so will only over-whelm an irritated stomach and cause her to throw everything back up.

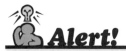

Alert!

Antidiarrheal medications that are made for adults, such as Imodium and Lomotil, are dangerous for children. Excessive doses of these medications can suppress normal breathing in children younger than two years old, and children have died from taking these medications. Pediatricians never recommend the use of these products for children with diarrhea caused by stomach viruses.

Once your child is able to drink water slowly, the next best thing is to offer some standard oral rehydration solution. Many commercial products will do the trick, but the one that tastes best is called Liquilyte. This is a standard rehydration solution made by Gerber, the famous baby food manufacturer. The well-known Pedialyte tastes horrible in comparison. (Try it yourself if you haven't lately. You'll find that it tastes pretty much like sea water, so don't be surprised if your child refuses Pedialyte.)

Juices and sport drinks like Gatorade or Powerade should be avoided. Even though they do provide fluid and some salt, they also contain too much sugar. Taking an excessive amount of these types of drinks can sometimes worsen and prolong diarrhea. Soft drinks are bad for the body at any time, and times of stomach problems are no exception.

Most physicians now recommend early reintroduction of solid foods to children with vomiting and diarrhea. Doing so shortens the course of the illness and prevents excessive weight loss. Numerous studies have shown that introduction of solids (including dairy products) does not induce more diarrhea or increase stool volume. For the same reason, if you're breast-feeding, you should continue to do so during the diarrheal episodes.

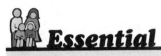
Essential

While it is a good idea to avoid high-fat foods, you should not withhold all food from a child with vomiting and diarrhea. If your child refuses solids, do not force him to eat. On the other hand, if he asks for solid foods, you should allow him to eat. Remember to offer small portions at first because his stomach will still be sensitive from the infection.

Pins and Needles

Many parents and doctors have developed the habit of using an intravenous solution to rehydrate any child who has dehydration, even if the dehydration is mild. People are jumping the gun by pulling out the needle and sticking children on a routine basis, even if these children could drink fluid by mouth. For this situation, the advancement of medical technology may actually be a disservice. Oral rehydration protocols used in developing countries are in fact a safer alternative to intravenous fluids.

Most parents regard IV hydration as a completely risk-free procedure, but this is far from the truth. The process of inserting a needle into a vein carries a small but real risk of infection, and pumping fluid directly into the vein can carry the risk of introducing air into the bloodstream. This could potentially be a dangerous situation.

If your child can drink fluid by mouth slowly and is not severely dehydrated, there is absolutely no need to put an IV into your child and load up the body with fluid via a needle. Even though IV fluid has its place in reversing severe dehydration, parents tend to put the pressure on the doctor to immediately resort to IV fluid or even hospitalization. When push comes to shove, some doctors might figure it's easier to give in to parental demand and carry out the unnecessarily invasive medical intervention.

To BRAT or Not to BRAT

Should your child avoid dairy products or milk when she has diarrhea? Theoretically, it sounds reasonable. Scientists know that the tissue responsible for digesting milk sugar is located on the surface of the intestine. During a diarrheal illness, the surface of the intestine gets somewhat damaged. In the past, physicians intuitively assumed that children's ability to digest milk during and after a diarrhea is impaired.

This may sound good on paper, but thank goodness that someone actually looked into this and tried to prove its validity. It turns out that this assumption is incorrect. In fact, those children who kept their diet pretty much the same during an episode of vomiting and diarrhea (including taking in dairy products) actually got better faster than those who had their diet restricted.

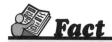 **Fact**

Babies who are drinking milk should stay on their usual milk when they have diarrhea. You should not dilute the formula or breast milk in any way during a diarrheal illness, and you should not feed your baby water until she is six months old.

The age-old wisdom of a BRAT (bread, rice, apple sauce, toast) diet in rehabilitating an irritated intestine has never had any scientific backing, yet doctors and nurses around the world still give this advice every day. Correcting the assumption that this is the best diet for a diarrheal child is a daunting task for a pediatrician, especially given that most parents at one time or another have heard this BRAT advice from a health professional. It is a great deal more difficult to discredit information that comes from a fellow health-care worker, and this old-school (and incorrect) way of thinking is ingrained in many parents' minds.

The best way to feed your diarrheal child is to continue his usual diet while excluding any fluids high in sugar (such as juice, soda, sport drinks). Unnecessarily restricting your child's diet during a bout of diarrhea is harmful.

Chronic Recurrent Abdominal Pain

Chronic recurrent abdominal pain is a common problem in pediatrics. Even though it is a harmless condition, it can be an overwhelming source of parental stress and anxiety. It is one of the most common reasons for visits to a general pediatric practice.

The official American Academy of Pediatrics definition of chronic recurrent abdominal pain requires the recurrent pain to have lasted for more than three months and to occur at least once a month. The pain is usually vague, but it can be quite intense, and it is not generally associated with eating.

The Many Faces of Pain

Your child may experience abdominal pain for many reasons. Some children have sensitive stomachs and are more prone to experience intestinal discomfort. Numerous triggers have been found to induce abdominal pain, including stresses at school, a diet high in fat and oil, and even migraines. The first step in solving your child's abdominal pain problem is a visit to your pediatrician.

The doctor will obtain a detailed history about your child's diet, bowel-movement patterns, any potential stresses in your child's life, changes in routines, and presence of intestinal disorders in other family members.

Abdominal pain that is caused by something benign should never wake a child up from sleep or cause any unintentional weight loss. Other warning signs that may indicate the presence of a serious medical condition include the following:

- Fever
- Blood in the stool
- Chronic diarrhea
- Persistent vomiting

If your child experiences abdominal pain along with any of these symptoms, you should seek medical attention immediately. In addition, if there are other members of your family who have serious gastrointestinal disorders, this should also prompt you to have your child checked sooner rather than later.

The Brain in the Belly

A growing body of scientific evidence points to a "functional" trigger as the cause of chronic abdominal pain in children. When your child suffers from abdominal pain, in other words, there isn't really anything "wrong," per se. Instead, it may be that your child's body is misinterpreting normal cues from the gut and signaling them as harmful or painful.

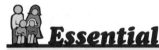 *Essential*

Just as the complex nervous system inside the brain can sometimes cause harmless headaches, the network of intestinal nerves can sometimes trigger pain in the belly. Even though some headaches can be the harbinger of something serious, most headaches are benign. This is also true for abdominal pains.

Unbeknownst to most people, the intestine is covered by a network of nerves so intricate and highly sophisticated that it rivals the complexity of the neuronal system inside the brain.

This intestinal nervous system can automate the digestive movement of the intestine independently of any controls from the brain. Not surprisingly, such a complicated system can sometimes misfire and interpret innocuous signals as harmful. This is what most scientists believe happens when a child experiences a functional pain from the intestine.

When food traverses the length of the intestinal tract, the pressure inside the intestine changes as a clump of food is squeezed from one segment to the next. Normally, most people do not sense this pressure change. For children with functional abdominal pain, however, the oversensitive nervous system in the intestines inappropriately registers this pressure change as pain. Even though nothing is really wrong with the digestive process, their body senses discomfort.

More Tests, Please

The responsibility of the parents and pediatricians is to differentiate the vast majority of children with functional abdominal pain from the minority with serious digestive illnesses. For the most part, the doctor can rule out most dangerous conditions simply by taking a comprehensive history from the child and the parents. The description and timing of the pain with other associated symptoms can exclude most serious medical conditions.

If the history alone is insufficient to exclude a dangerous cause for the abdominal pain, the doctor will order additional blood tests and a stool analysis. X rays are not a very useful means of diagnosing chronic abdominal pain, and they are seldom used in the workup.

Coping with Chronic Recurrent Abdominal Pain

After your pediatrician has reassured you that everything looks fine and the pain originates from an overly sensitive gut, what can you do to alleviate the pain? The pain is definitely real; it's not just in your child's head.

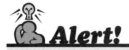
Alert!

It is important to maintain your child's routine despite the pain. Some children may try to take advantage of the situation and use the pain as an excuse to skip school or chores. As a parent, you cannot allow your child to benefit from this situation, or you might unknowingly prolong the situation.

Most experts generally recommend a diet high in fiber as a means of reducing the intensity and frequency of stomach pain. Lowering the amount of fat and oil your child eats can also help alleviate the pain. That's because oily substances in the gut slow down intestinal movement, which can worsen a functional pain.

Most functional abdominal pain can be managed with dietary modification alone. Medication use is discouraged; if it is prescribed, the managing physician must use it judiciously. Using medication may reinforce the idea that there is something wrong with the intestine, which is not the case for the vast majority of children with chronic abdominal pain.

Tackling Constipation

Constipation can occur in a child of any age. This section, however, focuses on the problem of constipation in toddlers. This tends to be a behavioral problem. A bad experience with the process of bowel movement is enough to trigger a chain of events that eventually leads to chronic constipation. Once the fall from grace occurs, it's all downhill from there, and that's not a pretty sight.

The First Hard Stool

It all begins with a single bad experience. A simple dietary change can harden your child's stool to the degree that passing the hard stool is an unpleasant experience. Your child is no fool. He will not only remember this bad experience, he will do the best he can to avoid having to go through it again. In fact, it's possible that he will seriously consider not having another bowel movement for the rest of his life.

Of course, everyone knows that would be impossible, but such a daunting goal would not faze a stubborn toddler. Every time he senses the need to have a bowel movement, he'll do everything within his power to avoid passing the stool. You will undoubtedly witness many of these valiant struggles. When the urge to defecate comes, you'll find your child suddenly drops everything that he's doing and stiffens up. He will remain motionless and may cross his legs to help discourage the stool from coming out. Sooner or later, the wave of contractions will pass, and he'll resume his normal activities.

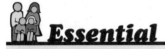 **Essential**

Infants less than a year old do not have the ability to willfully hold in stools. If your baby has hard stools, the best way to ameliorate the condition is to provide a small amount of diluted prune juice on a regular basis. Remember, babies can go for five to seven days without having a bowel movement, and this is considered to be normal as long as the stools are not hard.

This is the classic sign of constipation in children. Pediatricians refer to this as stool-withholding behavior. This behavior is the root of all evils, because it generates a cycle of pain and increasingly hardened stools. The task for the parents and the pediatricians is to break this relentless cycle of suffering.

The Initial Disimpaction

Once the vicious cycle of painful bowel movements and stool withholding is established, it must be broken one way or the other before your child can embark on the road to recovery. The first order of business is to eliminate all the hard stool that has been accumulating inside the intestine.

Of course, there is no way that your child is going to accomplish this willingly. After all, stool withholding is part of the problem, and logical reasoning with your toddler is usually futile.

Therefore, the only way this can be accomplished is by force. While this procedure doesn't have to be brutal, it is inevitably against the wish of your child, so a struggle is almost always guaranteed during this process.

The disimpaction can be accomplished in many ways. If a large bulky stool is stuck in the rectum, the doctor sometimes tries to disimpact the bulk by sticking a finger into the anus and manually remove the stool. If this is not feasible or not necessary, a large amount of gentle laxative or an enema can often do the trick.

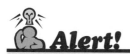

Alert!

Even though chronic constipation in a toddler is most likely caused by a behavioral problem, there are some rare but real medical conditions that can cause constipation. If your baby has had severe constipation since birth, or has other developmental delays, the constipation may be a manifestation of an underlying neurological problem (a condition called Hirschprung's disease).

The safest and most popular laxative for children is mineral oil. While there are other safe and effective alternatives, most pediatricians favor mineral oil because of its safety profile. The intestine cannot absorb this medicine, so even if your child ingests a large quantity of it, overdosing is practically impossible. The only thing that too much mineral oil can cause is excessive loose stool. But after all, isn't this the outcome you're shooting for when your child is constipated?

You may have to start with a repeat dose of mineral oil to empty the intestine of all the stool. Generally, it is a good idea to continue administering the mineral oil until what's coming out from the other end is colorless (neither brown nor yellow). Your pediatrician should advise you on the proper dosage, depending on the body size and age of your child.

Maintenance Treatment

After you have successfully cleaned out your child's intestine, the struggle against constipation has just begun. Getting a fresh start is only the beginning of the long and tedious process of treating constipation because the root of the problem is not resolved. Your child still fears going to the bathroom and having a bowel movement. In fact, after the torturous process of disimpaction with a laxative, your child probably has developed even more distaste for passing stools.

What parents must do at this stage is aim to keep the stool moving through the child's intestine without allowing it to be backed up. You can expect your child to actively fight against this goal because the fear of stooling still looms large over his head. Your job is to continue giving the mineral oil, usually at a smaller dosage than you did in the initial disimpaction phase, on a regular basis. You cannot allow your child to withhold stools again, or you'll be back at square one. Hopefully, after a few weeks your child will get used to the passage of soft stools and will stop trying to actively retain stools.

This maintenance phase may last for a long time, especially if your child has been suffering from constipation for quite a while. Once things are going well, you cannot grow complacent and slack off on the mineral oil treatments. Your child is at risk for a relapse for the first few months of the maintenance phase.

If your stop treatment prematurely, your child will stop passing stools and become constipated again.

High-Fiber Diet

You can never go wrong eating lots of fresh fruits and vegetables. There is a reason why everyone touts their virtues: Not only do they ward off childhood obesity, but they are an excellent source of fiber. There is also increasing scientific evidence that a diet rich in fresh fruits and vegetables can lower the risk of cancer development.

 Essential

Don't forget to increase your child's water intake while you're adding fiber to her diet. A diet high in fiber that does not also include an increased intake of water can actually worsen constipation instead of helping it. A high-fiber diet must be accompanied with a lot of water intake in order to maximize the benefit of the fiber in the intestine.

Fruits, vegetables, and beans are all excellent sources of fiber. Especially beneficial are pitted fruits, such as peaches, pears, and plums. Unbuttered popcorn is also a great and tasty source of fiber that most children love, and raisins also make a good snack for your child.

Even though increasing the amount of fiber and water in your child's diet is certainly an important aspect of treating constipation, the hardest part is changing your toddler's attitude about having bowel movements. It takes a tremendous amount of patience on the part of you and your child to correct the attitude. If you are determined to resolve this stubborn problem, you must be mentally prepared to be in it for the long haul.

CHAPTER 9

The Shot Heard Round the World

On its own, the topic of childhood immunization is controversial enough to fill an entire library with books on the subject. Since this book only has space for a single chapter, it will focus on the common misconceptions and fears about vaccines. An overwhelming abundance of vaccine opponents are always working hard to abolish childhood immunization. They tend to be more vocal and thereby to garner more media coverage than people who support the need for immunization. There is always a need for more authoritative medical sources to discredit the myths associated with the common medical procedure.

How Do Vaccines Work?

Before any meaningful exchange of information about the benefit and risk of vaccines can take place, parents must understand how vaccines protect children from infections. Vaccines are completely different from antibiotics. Antibiotics are prescribed to help fight a bacterial infection that has established itself inside the body. Vaccines prevent infections from establishing themselves in the first place. This makes vaccination a superior strategy in fighting infectious agents. After all, an ounce of prevention is worth more than a pound of cure.

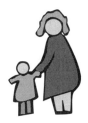

An FBI File

Giving your child a vaccine against a bad germ is equivalent to setting up an FBI file for that germ in your child's body. Most vaccines are made from bits and pieces of the bad germ. When your doctor gives your child a vaccine, it's like she's distributing flyers of the most-wanted bad germs all over your child's body.

After a vaccination, your child's immune system is alerted to the presence of a particular bad germ and is prepared to do battle against it if it ever appears in the body again. If that particular germ tries to infiltrate your child's immunologic defense, the immune system is alerted immediately. Before the bad germ can make any inroads, it is caught and exterminated. Vaccines in no way weaken the immune system. If anything, they empower your child's body in its defenses and beef up the border patrol against unauthorized germ invasion.

Booster Shots

The effect of most vaccines does not last forever. As the FBI file gets old, it tends to collect dust and get pushed behind some cabinet. Over a long period of time, it can even be lost or forgotten. The immune system's memory isn't perfect, and that's why your child often requires several booster shots for the same infectious agent. Getting these booster shots is just as important as getting the primary vaccine. You can't afford to have your child's immunity lose track of these dangerous bad guys.

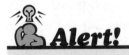

Don't forget that even adults need to get shots once in a long while. A tetanus booster is required periodically throughout life, once every ten years. If you are unsure when you got your last tetanus booster, check with your doctor. It's only fair for your child to get to see Daddy and Mommy get shots sometimes, too.

The boosters are typically scheduled at predetermined intervals. If they are given too early or too close together, the booster effect is not optimized. If the memory of a criminal germ is still fresh in the immune system's mind, it is a waste to provide the immune system with another reminder. Taking your child to the pediatrician at the instructed intervals is crucial in keeping your child's immune system as effective as possible.

Getting Sick from Shots

Many parents fear that a vaccination might make their child sick. While vaccinations can cause mild reactions in some children, these consequences are typically rare and minor. This is a fear that might still be lingering from decades ago, when vaccines were first developed. Children today are not administered the same vaccines that your grandfather was given many decades ago. The vaccines of today work better, and they have significantly fewer side effects. Overall, the advancement in vaccine production has rendered worries about illness as a result of vaccination obsolete.

Dead or Alive

Vaccines are usually formulated using a "killed" version of the infectious agent being vaccinated against. It is impossible to get the infection itself from this type of vaccine. Most vaccines fall into this category, and parents never have to worry about their children getting sick from the vaccine.

However, it is also true that a few vaccines, including vaccines for chickenpox, the measles, mumps, and rubella, are made using live viruses. The live viruses in these shots have been greatly weakened. While it is possible for these "live" vaccines to cause a very mild case of the infection, they cannot cause a normal infection. In other words, no one who is vaccinated against chickenpox gets chickenpox from the vaccine, though there is a small chance that the vaccination might cause a mild fever and a slight rash. No one becomes very ill from these live but weakened viruses.

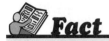 **Fact**

The polio vaccine used to have a live-virus formulation that could cause paralysis in very rare circumstances (literally one in a million). However, this type of vaccine has not been used in the United States since 1996. No one in the United States is giving out this form of the polio vaccine anymore.

One of the biggest rumors out there is that the flu shot will make you come down with the flu. It's unclear how this myth originated, but it has absolutely no scientific backing. Every year, the flu vaccine is formulated from particles of the various flu viruses in existence. This formulation can change, depending on which flu strain is most virulent and therefore most likely to make people sick. As a consequence, the flu vaccine does not contain a whole flu virus of any particular strain, alive or dead. There is therefore no way that the flu shot can make you catch the flu. A fear of catching the flu from the flu shot is like the fear of being run over by a pile of hubcaps.

It is true that some people might experience flu-like symptoms after the vaccine, but they are not getting sick from the flu. The difference is that the symptoms are very short-lived (lasting for a few hours), and they are mild. These feelings never cause any life-threatening complications that the flu virus itself can cause, such as pneumonia or a brain infection.

Weakened Immune System
Some parents worry that by using a vaccine to protect their child from an infection, they might be weakening the child's immune system. If the child can't get sick, they reason, the

immune system has no work to do. As a result, it might become too weak to fight off infections. It is impossible to vaccinate against every illness-causing virus on the planet. Consequently, a child's body is regularly exposed to plenty of infections that challenge the immune system and force it to stay strong and active.

On the other side of the coin, it is important to remember that the infections for which vaccines are now available were once considered dangerous. Chickenpox, for example, is not considered a serious illness today, but that is because children of recent generations have had the benefit of a vaccine against the disease. Children used to die from chickenpox before the vaccine became widespread. So while withholding a vaccine does force your child's immune system to work harder to fight off infection, there is always the chance that the infection will be too strong for a child's immature system to vanquish. Most children who get chickenpox do survive, but the process of getting a viral infection such as this is not benign. It's not a good idea to let your child get sick from an infection instead of protecting him with immunization.

Vaccines Your Child Needs

Vaccination standards are constantly changing. Even doctors can have a hard time keeping up with the latest recommendations made by the government and school districts. It's even harder for parents to keep abreast of all the shots their children need.

This section briefly covers the basics of each vaccine. For more extensive information, your doctor can provide you with a handout called the vaccine information sheet (or simply VIS). Request this from your doctor during each immunization visit.

Inevitably, by the time this book reaches the bookstore shelves, the following information will have changed. The best way to stay up to date on your child's vaccination needs is to communicate regularly with your pediatrician. Most doctors keep information on all the shots your child needs in the office.

DTaP Vaccine

This is a combination vaccine that consists of immunization against diphtheria, tetanus, and pertussis. Diphtheria is a respiratory infection that can cause heart and nerve damage in children. It is relatively rare now, after the vaccine initiative that started decades ago. Tetanus is a deadly bacterial infection that can be contracted from a contaminated wound. Once the infection is established, it is often fatal. Pertussis is commonly known as whooping cough. It causes a prolonged cough in older children and adults, but it can be deadly for infants. The "a" in DTaP stands for "acellular." It describes a new method in vaccine manufacturing. This combination vaccine is given four times, starting at the age of two months until the age of four.

A fifth booster shot has recently been introduced that is designed to protect adolescents from whooping cough and tetanus. Ask your teenager's doctor if she might need this booster.

IPV

This is the "inactivated" polio vaccine, which means that unlike the original polio vaccine, it contains no live polio virus. As a result of a successful childhood immunization program, polio has been effectively wiped out in developed countries. However, this vaccine is still necessary due to sporadic areas of outbreak around the world. Today's global travel makes it a distinct possibility that this virus could make a comeback if vaccination against it were halted. There are four total shots in this series of vaccine.

Hepatitis B Vaccine

Hepatitis B is mostly transmitted from pregnant or breast-feeding mothers to their babies. It can also be transmitted sexually and through blood transfusions. Hepatitis B is the number-one cause of liver failure in the world, and it causes the most liver cancer. There are three shots in this series.

Hepatitis A Vaccine

Even though hepatitis A is not as deadly as hepatitis B or C, it can still be debilitating. This infection is transmitted through contaminated foods. It's a frequent cause of dehydration and even hospitalization for travelers. A total of two shots is necessary to protect your child from this infection.

Hib Vaccine

Hib stands for "hemophilus influenza type b." It used to be a common cause of bacterial meningitis, which is a serious and often deadly infection of the brain. This bacterium can also cause pneumonia and another infection involving the back of the throat. Infections from this bacterium have become increasingly rare now, due to the effective protection offered by this vaccine. There are four shots in this vaccine series.

Pneumococcal Vaccine

Pneumococcus is a bacterium that commonly causes infection of the brain and lungs. It is also a common cause of blood infection and ear infection. Since the introduction of this vaccine, brain infection resulting from this bacterium has become rare. There are five shots in this series.

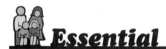 *Essential*

Don't forget that your child's pediatrician is the best source of information about immunization. If you have any concerns about vaccine safety, don't hesitate to open a discussion with your doctor. Pediatricians are trained health advocates, and they are happy to inform parents on the virtues of immunization as well as the possible side effects.

MMR Vaccine
MMR stands for "measles, mumps, and rubella." All three used to be common viral infections in children, but this vaccine has dramatically reduced the number of children afflicted with these infections. There are two shots in this series.

The Chickenpox Shot
Obviously, this vaccine is designed to protect children from chickenpox. Until recently, only one shot was recommended for most children. Extensive research has shown that a second booster may be necessary to more effectively protect children from this infection. The two shots need to be administered at least two months apart.

Tetanus Booster
The tetanus booster is given once every ten years to everyone, including adults. If your adolescent is over the age of eleven and has not had a tetanus shot in the last five years, it's time for him to get this booster. Starting in 2005, a whooping cough vaccine component was added to the tetanus booster for adolescents. It's called the Tdap (not to be confused with DTaP).

Meningococcal Vaccine
This is a new vaccine introduced in 2006. Meningococcal infection is a life-threatening infection that is common among older teens. It can be rapidly progressive, killing its victim in less than twenty-four hours after the first sign of infection. As a result, this vaccine is recommended for all teenagers, starting from age eleven.

The Rotavirus Vaccine
The rotavirus vaccine was introduced toward the end of 2006. It protects infants from rotavirus, which causes severe vomiting and diarrhea. Even though this infection is usually not

deadly, it is perhaps one of the most common causes of dehydration and hospitalization for infants during the winter.

This vaccine is given orally in a liquid form. There are a total of three doses for this vaccine.

HPV Vaccine

HPV stands for "human papilloma virus." Certain strains of this virus are believed to contribute to the development of cervical cancer. It is recommended that girls from the age of nine to twenty-six get this vaccine. There are three shots in the series.

The recommendation for this vaccine has generated much controversy because it protects children from a sexually transmitted disease. Some groups claim that this vaccine encourages adolescents to behave promiscuously, but most parents are receptive to this vaccine.

Mercurial Science

One of the main objections that vaccine opponents have to childhood immunization has to do with the presence of mercury in vaccines. However, since March 2001, mercury has been virtually eliminated from childhood vaccines. With the exception of the flu vaccine, none of the childhood vaccines administered to patients under the age of six years contains mercury as a preservative. What most critics of vaccinations fear no longer exists.

Historical Tragedy

Until 2001, some pediatric vaccines were manufactured with mercury. At high doses, mercury is a known neurotoxin, which means that it can cause brain damage if someone is exposed to large quantities of it. So why in the world would anyone put mercury in children's vaccines in the first place?

Back in 1928, twelve children died from a severe bacterial infection caused by a contaminated bottle of vaccine. After this tragedy, it was clear that something needed to be done about the possibility of vaccine bottle contamination. Consequently, a small amount of mercury-based preservative was added to some vaccines to hinder bacterial growth. It was used in extremely minute quantity, and it was considered innocuous to human health. The preservative appeared to work well, as there were no more cases of children dying from bacterially contaminated vaccines.

A Turning Point

In 1997, as a broader control measure aimed at minimizing mercury levels in all food and drugs, the FDA conducted a study of the mercury content of vaccines for childhood diseases. Until that time, vaccines with mercury preservative had been given to millions of children for decades with no apparent ill effects.

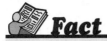 **Fact**

In 1997, the FDA issued a recommendation that all traces of mercury be removed from childhood vaccines by 2001. The new recommendation was not made out of any recent evidence that harm had resulted from the use of mercury. Instead, the recommendation was made because health officials were concerned that parents might refuse vital immunizations for their children out of an unfounded fear of mercury toxicity.

Even if your child received vaccinations prior to 2001, there is no reason to be alarmed. Aside from a mild allergic reaction to the preservative, no one was ever harmed by the minuscule quantity of mercury in those vaccines. And if your child was born after 2001, you don't have to worry about mercury in vaccines at all.

While some flu vaccines still contain mercury as a preservative, 8 million mercury-free doses of the flu vaccines were available in 2005 in the United States. So if you are still worried, you can specifically request a mercury-free flu vaccine from your doctor. The FDA is currently working with the vaccine manufacturers to get rid of all mercury-containing flu vaccines.

Common Vaccine Reactions

The vaccines available today are a lot less likely to cause any side effects than those administered generations ago. Still, it is possible for some reaction to occur in a minority of children. The vast majority of these reactions are minor and brief. It is exceedingly rare for a vaccine-triggered reaction to require medical intervention.

Fever

Fever is by far the most common vaccine-related reaction in children. It can happen with the first set of vaccinations, or it can happen with subsequent booster shots. Children of all ages are susceptible to this reaction. It is estimated that less than 10 percent of children receiving vaccinations will get a fever. The number may be higher or lower, depending on the vaccine.

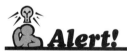

Alert!

Many infants become irritable after certain vaccines, particularly with the combination vaccine that protects against tetanus and the whooping cough (DTaP). This reaction is not expected to be prolonged. If your child remains irritable for more than three hours after the vaccination or cries continuously for more than an hour, contact your doctor immediately.

Regardless of how high the temperature, the fever usually doesn't last for more than three days. If it does, call your doctor for an appointment to have your child evaluated. There might be another cause for the fever.

If your child's temperature is less than 104°F and transient (or changing), you can administer acetaminophen (Tylenol) to your child to make him more comfortable. Please refer to Chapter 5 for additional advice on fever management.

Local Skin Reaction

Skin redness at the site of injection and rash are common vaccine reactions. They generally do not cause any discomfort for the child, and most of them disappear in less than three days.

However, the vaccine that protects against tetanus and whooping cough (DTaP) is notorious for its tendency to cause a large, red bump under the skin at the injection site. This reaction is especially common after the fourth or fifth vaccination in the DTaP series (which is usually given at the time your child enters kindergarten).

If your child develops a mildly tender bump at the site of a vaccination, don't panic. The vast majority of cases are not caused by infection or a serious allergic reaction. The area of redness may be quite large (larger than an inch is not unusual), but the pain is generally minor. The discomfort should not prevent your child from using the arm or the leg. If the pain is intense or if it prevents your child from walking or using his arm, you should seek medical attention.

The Link to Autism

Even though no association between autism and any childhood vaccine has ever been scientifically established, many parents hold this firm conviction. Despite statements made by prestigious and trustworthy groups like the American Academy of Pediatrics and the American Medical Association, many parents would rather listen to activist groups and people without any medical credentials. It is even more ironic that most of these parents tend to be more educated than the general public.

Bad Timing

Before embarking on an examination of the relationship between autism and the measles-mumps-rubella (MMR) vaccine, it is first necessary to clarify a basic point of logic. A temporal association (that is, an association in time, when one thing follows another) is not the same as a causal relationship (that is, a cause-and-effect relationship, when one thing causes something else to happen). To explain this further, here's an examination of a phenomenon that is unrelated to vaccination or autism.

We all know that road traffic tends to be heaviest during the morning and evening rush hours, when people are commuting to and from work. It is also true to say that traffic is most congested when the sun is rising and when it is going down. That means we can accurately predict that traffic jams will occur at around the time of sunrise and sunset. Would it be logical to state that the sun therefore has some mysterious influence on the flow of traffic? Or could we say that heavy traffic causes the sun to rise or set? This is obviously not the case. Just because the two events happen at around the same time, it does not follow that there is any temporal association between the two—that is, one does not necessarily trigger the other.

The argument that some scientists initially used to propose the alleged link between the MMR vaccine and autism was based on a similar temporal association. The MMR vaccine is usually administered right after a child turns one year old. Most cases of autism are first diagnosed at around this time. It is not uncommon for parents of autistic children to recall that things first started going wrong immediately after the administration of the MMR vaccine.

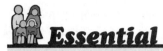 **Essential**

> Autism is a brain disorder that hinders a person's ability to interpret sensory input and to communicate with others. One of the key features of autism is speech delay. Because this prominent feature of autism does not manifest itself until the age of one, when speech is typically acquired, it is difficult to make a diagnosis of autism prior to that age.

Many vaccine opponents argue that autism must be caused by vaccination rather than a genetic component. If autism was an inherited condition—that is, something the child was born with—wouldn't it make sense for some behavioral problems to surface before the age of one? In order for this argument to hold water, children affected by autism should show no signs of the disorder prior to receiving the MMR vaccine. As investigation into the causes of autism has become more sophisticated, it has become clear that this prediction is false.

Child development experts are now able to identify children with autistic traits at an earlier and earlier age. Most autistic children manifest some subtle behavioral abnormalities before they are six months old. Many of the developmental clues are difficult to detect unless they are monitored by a pediatric developmental expert, but they are present nevertheless.

If signs of autism manifest themselves earlier than a year, why are most cases of autism diagnosed *after* that age? This is because these signs may be so mild that even the most experienced parents can overlook them. Major developmental problems, such as speech delay, do not become apparent until after children have become old enough to acquire speech.

The bottom line is that the temporal association between the MMR vaccine and autism does not indicate a causal relationship. Just because autism is often diagnosed right after the MMR vaccine is administered doesn't mean that the vaccine triggered the condition. In fact, causal relationship between the vaccine and autism has been repeatedly refuted by many clinical studies.

The Rise of Autism

There are more children with autism today than ever before. This is true even after taking population growth into consideration. Some experts believe that this increase in the number of cases is due to increased reporting. Doctors are more able to diagnose and subsequently report autistic cases to the national database than they were twenty years ago, and this undoubtedly contributes to the overall increase in the number of diagnosed autistic cases. However, most behavioral experts believe that this increased reporting does not completely account for the recent rise of autism.

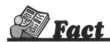

Fact

Despite extensive research, experts still do not know the cause of autism, but it's clear that there is a definite genetic predisposition. Siblings of autistic children have a one-in-twenty chance of having autism themselves. This is significantly higher than the risk found in the general population.

Unfortunately, it was just as the reported cases of autism were rising that the MMR vaccine was introduced. The fact of the matter is that even though the percentage of children getting the MMR vaccine has not changed significantly over the past ten years, the percentage of children being diagnosed with autism continues to rise. If the MMR vaccine were truly to blame for triggering autism, the rate of autism diagnosis should have remained stable as well. This is not the case.

Lack of Causality

Despite numerous studies attempting to ascertain a causal link between the MMR vaccine and autism, no such relationship has been established. Since no one really knows what truly causes autism, it is impossible to either prove or disprove any hypothesis at this point. However, one thing is certain: If the general population stops receiving the MMR vaccine, a massive outbreak of measles, mumps, and rubella is destined to occur. All three diseases used to kill and disable thousands of children each year before the introduction of this vaccine, and the MMR vaccine has saved millions of children already. Turning back the clock and not immunizing children is simply out of the question.

Some vaccine opponents advocate the practice of separating out each component of this combination vaccine to prevent autism. There is absolutely no scientific evidence that this practice make any difference. However, it does make it exceedingly difficult for children to get these vaccines independently. Most commercial manufacturers stopped making separate vaccines decades ago, and most medical offices do not stock these separated vaccines. The logistical nightmare of obtaining these vaccines just means that your child will fall behind on her vaccinations, which puts her at a higher risk of contracting these dangerous infections.

CHAPTER 10

Rash Decision

S kin problems constitute a significant part of any pediatric practice. There are literally thousands of conditions that can affect the skin of your child. It would be impossible to attempt to go over every single one of them. In order to convey any useful information to the reader, this chapter focuses on only a few of the most common skin conditions in children.

Eczema

Eczema can be simply described as skin allergy. It is called atopic dermatitis in medical lingo, and it is actually a part of a large spectrum of allergic conditions that affect children. Two other conditions—nasal allergy and asthma—are discussed in Chapters 14 and 15. Together, these three conditions are known as the "atopic triad" because they are so closely related.

Itchy and Scratchy
Even though eczema is an allergic condition, most children with eczema do not have specific food allergies that trigger the skin outbreaks. Instead, the most common trigger for eczema is dryness. The trouble almost always starts when the skin gets dry.

The best way to understand this skin condition is to learn how a skin rash progresses. The initial trigger for the rash occurs when the skin becomes

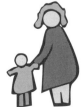

too dry. For someone without eczema, this would not be a big deal, but eczema sufferers experience an intense itch when the skin dries up. Children with eczema tend to have drier skin to begin with, so they are more prone to itchiness.

Once the itching starts, it's just a matter of time before the child starts to scratch the skin incessantly. This scratching causes damage to the surface of the skin, which leads to redness and rawness. This is the appearance of a typical eczema rash. The presence of this intense itch is mandatory for the development of eczema.

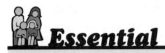 **Essential**

The entire cycle can be characterized as starting with dry skin. The dry skin itches, and the child scratches. Scratching the itch causes redness, which leads to infection. In order to alleviate eczema, the itch-scratch cycle must be broken. Breaking this cycle is the cornerstone of a successful eczema-management plan, and the best place to break the cycle is at the initial dryness stage.

If the scratching continues unabated, the skin surface can become raw and damaged. Once the skin surface is disrupted, bacteria on the surface of the skin can penetrate the damaged skin and cause a skin infection. Skin infection is the most serious problem facing children with severe eczema. Sometimes an untreated skin infection can evolve into a system-wide infection in the body.

Eczema can affect any part of the body, but depending on the patient's age, it is more likely to appear in different areas. For most infants, the face, ears, and neck are the areas most likely to be targeted by eczema. As your child grows older, the distribution of eczema tends to shift. School-age children are most likely going to have eczema in their elbows, behind the knees, in the armpits, and on the wrists. The skin around the eyes remains a popular spot for eczema. Adolescents and adults tend to have eczema on their hands.

Other factors, such as emotional stress, changes in humidity, and excessive sweating can also trigger eczema. Eczema tends to worsen during certain seasons. For most people suffering from eczema, skin condition frequently worsens during the winter and improves during the summer (assuming the weather is not too hot).

Breaking the Cycle

Since dryness is the first step of the itch-scratch cycle, it is most effective to stop the cycle at this early stage. Keeping the skin moist is essential. If you can successfully prevent your child's skin from getting too dry, you can avoid most eczema flare-ups.

There are many skin-care strategies that can be used to maintain skin moisture. Avoiding prolonged exposure to water and harsh soaps is a key step. Even though it is not absolutely necessary for children with eczema to avoid taking a bath, taking a shower is generally a better idea. In addition, keep the time spent in the shower as short as possible—ideally under ten minutes. Prolonged soaking of the skin with water washes away the natural skin oil and in the process dries out the skin.

If the weather is cool and your child does not get too dirty during the day, you might want to consider making bath or shower time less frequent—every other day, for instance, instead of daily. Even if your child becomes sweaty or dirty, try to consolidate all the washing to just once daily. Multiple showers in one day can excessively dry the skin and worsen eczema.

Using a harsh soap (such as Lever 2000) has the same effect as frequent washing; it deprives the skin of its natural moisture content. The best types of soap to use for children with eczema are those that include a moisturizer (such as Dove). In fact, if you can manage to get your child clean without using any soap at all, that's even better.

Since avoiding skin dryness is the foundation of controlling eczema, skin moisturizers have a critical role in keeping eczema attacks at bay. Cheap over-the-counter moisturizers are just as effective as the expensive ones sold at cosmetic counters. In fact, petroleum jelly works well for many children. The best time to apply a moisturizer is immediately after a shower. Moisturizing right after a shower helps to trap the water from the wash into the skin. Waiting too long allows that water to evaporate.

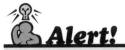

Alert!

A good rule of thumb to remember when purchasing moisturizers is that lotions are generally dispensed from a pump. Moisturizing creams or ointments are usually too thick to be pumped out, so they are sold in jars or small tubs with twist-off lids. You can't usually go wrong with buying a moisturizer in a jar.

Even though the brand name of the skin moisturizer is not important, you should only use a cream or a thick ointment for the job of moisturizing the skin. Lotions contain mostly water, and once the water content evaporates, the skin is left unprotected. In fact, some eczema may even get worse with repeated application of lotion.

Topical Medications

The powerful ability of steroids to subdue inflammation makes these medications the most effective treatment for eczema by far. Just a few days after using these medications, you will notice a drastic improvement in your child's eczema. These steroid medications are directly applied on the skin, and they come in either creams or ointments. Most topical steroids are prescribed by doctors, but some extremely weak ones can be purchased over the counter.

However, you cannot apply topical steroids indiscriminately, which is the reason they must be used under the supervision of doctors. If these medicated creams and ointments are used too long or too often, they can cause the skin to become abnormally thin or to lose its natural pigmentation. Despite their efficacy, they must not be abused.

A new class of prescription creams for eczema came onto the market approximately ten years ago. These creams do not contain steroids, so they don't come with the same possible side effects. Examples in this class of medication include Protopic and Elidel.

These medications do not work nearly as well as steroids, and they tend to work a lot more slowly than topical steroids. Even though these medications do not thin out or bleach the skin like steroids, recent research suggests that they might increase the risk of skin cancer. This is obviously a worrisome finding, and more studies are needed to confirm this initial suspicion.

Anti-Itch Campaign

This is the aspect of eczema management that tends to be underutilized by physicians. Given that the itch-scratch cycle is the foundation for the formation of the eczema, it makes intuitive sense that if the itching can be prevented, the rash will also be a lot better. This is indeed the case.

 Essential

You can reduce the skin damage that results from scratching by keeping your child's fingernails short and trimmed. Short fingernails not only cause less trauma to the surface of the skin, they also tend to trap less dirt and bacteria. This may reduce the risk of getting a skin infection from the scratching.

The most effective medication to relieve itching is the oral antihistamine. Medications such as Claritin, Benadryl, and Atarax belong to this category. While using these medications, keep in mind that some of them can be sedating.

Long-Term Outlook

Fortunately, you can almost always count on the fact that your child's eczema will improve with age. Most children suffer significantly less from their eczema by the time they reach adolescence. Exactly when your child might start experiencing relief is difficult to predict. Some children start getting better by school age, and many others carry their eczema into adulthood.

Furthermore, eczema is a genetic condition. This means that if your child has eczema, the chance of your grandchildren suffering from eczema, asthma, and nasal allergy is significantly increased. Since you can't choose your parents, the only thing you can do is be vigilant and bring your child to the doctor at the earliest sign of a problem.

Chickenpox

Before the advent of a chickenpox vaccine ten years ago, chickenpox used to be a sort of rite of passage for almost all children. Even after widespread childhood vaccinations, chickenpox still exists in the community, although on a much smaller scale. With effective community immunization programs, chickenpox is fast becoming a rarity. This reduction in cases makes many new parents unfamiliar with this once-ubiquitous disease.

Most Contagious

The chickenpox virus is one of the most contagious agents known to scientists. Simply breathing near an affected person can make a susceptible individual sick. Direct physical contact is not required for transmission.

If you suspect that your child has chickenpox, contact your doctor for an appointment. If your doctor confirms the diagnosis of chickenpox, you'll have to isolate your child from other children to prevent an outbreak. Make prior arrangements with the doctor's office so your child does not spend half an hour in a waiting room full of babies. Most medical offices can accommodate patients with extremely contagious conditions. You may have to enter the office through a side or back door and be examined in a separate room.

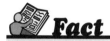 **Fact**

> After a child is exposed to chickenpox, it may take up to three weeks before she comes down with the rash. A child with chickenpox may transmit the virus to another child before the appearance of any rash. The unpredictability of the contagious period makes infection control especially difficult for chickenpox.

If your child has been exposed to chickenpox, it's not too late to act. Studies have shown that a vaccination given three to five days after the exposure can still be effective in reducing the severity of chickenpox. Call your doctor immediately if you believe your child has been exposed.

Bug Bites or Chickenpox

The chickenpox rash looks like small pimples and blisters on the body. It can occur anywhere from head to toe, sparing no area. It can be difficult to tell the difference between extensive insect bites on the body and a case of chickenpox. This is especially true since the advent of the chickenpox vaccine because a severe and extensive chickenpox rash is now less common. Children who contract chickenpox after they have been vaccinated sometimes just develop a few spots on their bodies.

Pediatricians try to distinguish between a mild chickenpox and bug bites by examining the location of the rash. If the rash only occurs on the exposed regions of the body, and it's known that the child has just returned from a week of camping next to a river, insect bites are the more likely culprit. On the other hand, if spots occur even on areas of the skin that are well protected, chickenpox is the more likely cause.

Taking Care of Your Child

If your child comes down with chickenpox, you can soothe her skin with oatmeal baths and lotions. To relieve the itching, you can use oral antihistamines such as Benadryl. Trim her nails short so that she doesn't cause too much damage to her skin when she scratches; scratched chickenpox blisters almost invariably scar.

One thing you should never do is give your child aspirin. If she has a fever, you can reduce her temperature with acetaminophen or ibuprofen. Administering aspirin to your child during chickenpox is associated with a lethal condition called Reye's syndrome. This condition causes swelling in the brain, and liver failure.

As a general rule of thumb, avoid using aspirin in anyone younger than the age of eighteen. Some children with heart problems and other rare conditions are required to take aspirin. Your pediatrician will advise you what to do if your child belongs to this small population.

Scabies

The mere mention of the word "scabies" is often enough to trigger a crawling sensation over anyone's body. Even though this condition has much social stigma attached to it, compared with conditions like asthma and diabetes it is not a serious condition.

Bugs with Eight Legs

Scabies is an intensely itchy condition that can affect people of all ages. Adults are certainly not immune, so if your child contracts scabies, you do have to worry about your own well-being. Fortunately, scabies is not as contagious as many other infectious diseases. It usually requires prolonged skin-to-skin contact to be transmitted from one person to another.

Scabies is caused by a microscopic bug that literally sets up residence inside your skin. An adult bug cannot survive for more than one day once it's detached from your skin. Your skin provides it with shelter and sustenance. It eats, poops, and has sex right under your skin. These bugs must feed on your skin constantly. If the thought of that doesn't make your skin crawl, not many things will.

The itch caused by scabies is intense. Not many other skin conditions other than eczema cause an itch whose intensity is enough to keep a child (and the parent) up all night scratching. Both of these conditions can cause a chronic itch. If multiple family members are itching at the same time, the culprit for the itching is very likely going to be scabies.

Pest Control

From a patient's perspective, it is more important to relieve the itching immediately than to get rid of the bugs. In fact, the intense itching may last up to six weeks after all the scabies parasites are dead. The residual allergic reaction to the dead bugs and their feces is the reason for the protracted itching.

Treating scabies requires a tremendous amount of patience. The physician must inform the parents when initiating therapy what to expect. A realistic expectation at the onset of treatment can prevent the parents from getting frustrated with the experience. Since scabies is contagious, every household member should be treated with the medication, even the ones who are not scratching.

Even though the resolution of itching takes so long, the actual bugs are fairly easy to kill. Apply the prescription cream all over your child's body from the neck down when your child goes to bed. Make sure you cover every inch of skin with the medication. Any area of skin that is missed could harbor a renegade bug, which could start a fresh infestation all over again. Usually a single treatment with a prescription cream obliterates all the bugs and their eggs. If there are infants under the age of one year in the household, ask your pediatrician for exact instructions on how to treat them.

Even as the scabies bugs are on their deathbed, your child will continue to experience the same intense itching. Antihistamine taken by mouth can offer significant relief from the suffering. You can administer antihistamine around the clock to make your child comfortable, but keep in mind that most of these medications cause drowsiness.

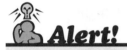

Alert!

The permethrin cream used to treat scabies is actually a neurotoxin. It disrupts the brain of these little bugs so that they cannot move or stay on the skin. This is also the reason that you should not apply this cream to your child repeatedly. One treatment is good, but four consecutive treatments may be harmful to your child. Follow the doctor's instructions exactly. Do not use the medication over and over again.

Beside antihistamine, steroid creams (the same ones that are used to treat eczema) are also beneficial. These creams reduce the skin irritation caused by the incessant scratching, but they do not work as fast as the oral antihistamines.

Point of No Return

After killing off all the parasites on the skin, your work is not quite finished. Scabies bugs may be hiding in clothing and bed sheets. It is critical to launder all the clothes worn on the day before the treatment as well as all the bed sheets and to cycle them for at least an hour in the dryer afterward. Anything that cannot be tossed into the washer can be placed inside a sealed trash bag for two weeks. It takes up to ten days for the scabies eggs to hatch, and scabies parasites cannot survive without feeding on human skin for more than a day. If either the eggs or scabies bugs are trapped in a bag for two weeks, they will all be dead.

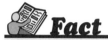 **Fact**

Contrary to many beliefs, human scabies are not transmitted from pets or to pets. Therefore, leave your lovely animals alone when you treat everyone in the household for scabies. Do not blame them for the infestation or treat them with scabicide. They are just innocent bystanders.

It is generally unnecessary to spray pesticide or treat carpets, the upholstery of sofas, and other furniture. Since scabies parasites cannot survive long unless they are on the human skin, they do not willingly leave it.

Burning Questions

Burns are a significant cause of hospitalization and even permanent disability for children. Thousands of children suffer every year from severe burns that require medical attention, and almost all of these can be prevented one way or the other. Successful burn prevention not only requires vigilance on the part of parents and caretakers, but it also relies on preventative measures implemented around the house to segregate toddlers from hot objects in the first place.

Accidents Happen

Despite the best of intentions and precautions, children regularly suffer from burns caused by hot liquids and surfaces.

Children are naturally curious, and during the process of exploring the exciting new world, it's almost inevitable that they will suffer minor burns at one time or another.

The first thing you should do after your child is burned is to remove your child from the source of heat to prevent any additional burn. Immediately run cold water over the burned skin and keep it submerged as long as possible (half an hour or more). The cold water keeps the heat on the surface of the skin from penetrating deeper into the tissue. As you drench the skin with cold water, remove any jewelry or clothing from the burned area. These objects can trap heat and cause deeper burns into the skin.

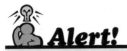

Alert!

A common old wives' tale instructs parents to treat a burn by smearing the affected skin with butter. Doing so only makes a burn worse. The grease from the butter traps heat against the skin, making the tissue damage deeper and more serious. Do not apply anything on the surface of the skin immediately after a burn.

After the burn cools down, take a look at the skin. If the skin starts to form blisters, you need to contact your doctor for a visit. If your child suffers a burn on the face, in the genital area, or over a large area of the body (larger than the palm of your hand), you should seek medical attention without delay. If the burn is mild and does not require a doctor's visit, you can treat the skin with a moisturizing cream. If the skin blisters or breaks open at any time, you should take your child to the pediatrician.

Rising Sun

Inadequate sun protection is a rampant phenomenon in children. Adults often neglect to protect themselves and their children from the sun. Even if sunscreen is applied prior to sun exposure, it is often done insufficiently. The sunscreen is often applied only once, at the beginning of the day, and forgotten. This creates a problem because as children sweat and engage in active play, the sunscreen is gradually removed. It is especially important to reapply sunscreen if children are engaged in water activities.

 Essential

Babies under six months old are too young to use sunscreens. Their skin is so sensitive that the application of sunscreen might trigger an allergic reaction. What parents must do is to shield their tender skin from the sun. Even brief sun exposure can result in a serious sunburn.

Parents commonly want to know what type of sunscreen they should use. An SPF rating of at least 15 is mandatory to protect the skin, and an SPF higher than 45 is usually overkill. Remember, reapplication is the key, not a high SPF number. If your child is swimming or sweating a lot, you need to reapply the sunscreen at least every two hours.

Even with meticulous use of sunscreen, the best way to protect your child from skin damage is with a layer of clothing or another physical barrier. Large-brimmed hats and umbrellas are more effective than any sunscreen if they can shield your child's skin completely.

Warts

Warts are nothing more than a minor skin infection caused by a common virus. It holds no more mystical power than the viruses that cause the common cold. As a virus, it can be passed from one person to another. What is annoying about this virus is that it tends to cause warts for extremely long period of time, and there is no quick and easy way to get rid of them. It's not uncommon for some children to suffer from warts for many years.

Managing parent expectation is one of the pediatrician's most important roles. Even though there are numerous ways to treat warts, none of them is satisfactorily effective. Most methods of treatment require multiple visits to the doctor's office. You must keep this in mind at the onset of therapy, or you will end up extremely dissatisfied and frustrated.

Over-the-Counter Wart Removers

The basic idea behind treating warts is to remove the wart-infected skin along with the wart virus. All treatments involve some way of getting rid of skin. Warts can often be successfully removed using over-the-counter wart remedies. These come in the form of acidic liquids, stickers, and scrubs. Usually it is a good idea to try the bandages or stickers first because these treatments do not cause any pain.

Cryotherapy

Cryotherapy is the use of extreme cold to induce localized frostbite on the skin and destroy the skin along with the warts. The first thing your pediatrician will do is warn you that this treatment is excruciating. It's no exaggeration. Your child is not acting up or making a scene when he screams as if he were suffering from medieval torture. It is that painful. Parents must take this into consideration when offered this treatment option.

Despite the pain, it usually requires multiple rounds of cryotherapy before the warts disappear. This means that you have to bring your child back over and over again for this type of torture. No one said treating warts is fun, and this is the reason many pediatricians prefer the more humane method of wart management.

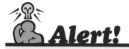
Alert!

After cryotherapy, the frostbitten skin can form a large blood blister. The appearance of it can be alarming to parents. If a blister forms, do not intentionally pop it. Leave it alone. If it breaks by itself, you can apply a topical antibiotic ointment to it to prevent infection.

Surgical Removal

Surgical removal of warts is fast and relatively painless, but this type of surgery can only be performed by a dermatologist. Most pediatricians do not have the proper equipment or schedule to surgically remove warts, which means that you will need a separate appointment with a specialist to seek this option. Keep in mind that even surgery is not a foolproof way of getting rid of warts once and for all. Warts frequently return, and additional surgical removal is required.

Molluscum

This is a type of skin condition that is different from the typical wart, but the best way to think of molluscum is that it is the cousin of the typical wart. It is also caused by a virus, and it is also contagious by touch. However, this virus tends to affect different areas of the body than the typical wart. Instead of being concentrated on the fingers and hands, this virus can affect exposed skin all over the body. It is not uncommon for molluscum to occur on children's faces, which is most unfortunate.

Similar to the common wart, molluscum is purely a cosmetic annoyance. The virus does not penetrate deep into the skin. The appearance of the lesion is different from typical warts as well. Molluscum bumps look like little round drops of dew collecting on the skin. They are very small, usually only slightly bigger than the period at the end of this sentence. They often occur in clusters. Sometimes they can have a small dimple in the center of the bump.

Some children find them irritating and itchy. In fact, molluscum bumps may take on a different appearance because the affected child has scratched the original rash beyond recognition.

The treatment for molluscum is similar to that for warts. Molluscum bumps tend to be more contagious than the common wart, which makes prevention of scratching even more important for this condition.

Pimples

The pimple is literally a symbol of youthfulness. Pimples are triggered by raging hormones and improper skin care. A combination of factors triggers the origin of acne, but the first step is the plugging of skin pores. The pores are plugged up by the material produced by the skin itself. Once the openings of these pores are blocked, the pores themselves swell up with the accumulation of secretions, and bacteria start to flourish inside these puffed-up pores. This is the simplified story of pimples.

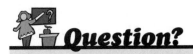 **Question?**

Do certain foods worsen acne?
Dermatologists used to believe that acne was not connected to diet, but recent research has revealed that a diet high in refined sugar drastically increases a person's chance of developing acne. Cultures that do not have any refined sugar in their diet have never heard of the acne condition or dental cavities.

Emotional stress affects acne outbreak because stress can modify hormone level. In turn, the hormone encourages the production of sticky material in the skin, thereby allowing more pores to be clogged. Let your teenager know that staying calm is a good strategy for preventing acne from forming.

Treating acne, once again, is about managing expectation. It often takes six to eight weeks before significant improvement can be appreciated. Make sure your child understands this when embarking upon a treatment regimen. Otherwise, you'll end up with an adolescent who has even more angst.

Benzoyl Peroxide

Benzoyl peroxide is the most popular initial acne treatment for many reasons. It is available over the counter, and it does not have any serious side effects. It should be applied right after the skin is cleaned. Some people can develop an allergic reaction to it, so it's wise to use it sparingly at first.

Antibiotics

Antibiotics can be used topically or taken orally. Both methods are effective in ameliorating acne. Topical application causes fewer side effects, but the oral form generally works better. Your doctor will decide the best form of treatment for your child.

Vitamin-A Derivatives

These medications, commonly known as retinoid or Accutane, can be extremely helpful in controlling acne. However, they carry significant health risk if used improperly. Particularly, the oral form of these medications can cause serious birth defects if a female user becomes pregnant while taking it.

Pediatricians and general practitioners usually do not prescribe the oral form of these medications themselves. The use of retinoid is best monitored by a dermatologist.

CHAPTER 11

Treating Scrapes and Cuts

As long as there are playful children who like to climb trees and run around fearlessly, there will be no shortage of "ouchies" that accompany their stunts. Almost all the time, parents can handle such minor injuries themselves without seeking the help of medical professionals. However, parents don't always know the best way to manage these injuries. Occasionally, a failure to do the right thing will do nothing worse than prolong the healing process. Other measures, however, can worsen the wound and cause infections.

Steps of Healing

Your child's skin may seem soft and tender to you, but it's an intimidating fortress wall to germs. Without this extremely effective barrier against the elements and invading germs, your child would be at great risk of suffering from dehydration and life-threatening infections. When this natural barrier is breached on a large scale, such as with burn patients, life-threatening complications can quickly develop.

Fortunately, extensive skin trauma isn't nearly as common as the minor cuts and scrapes your child experiences. Whenever this external defense is compromised, even in the case of a minor cut, the body immediately tries to repair the injury because it recognizes the urgency of such a breach in security.

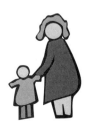

Small Construction Workers

The human body is truly a miraculous thing. One of its most amazing qualities is its ability to repair and heal itself. Even though machines are tougher and stronger for many tasks, none of them has this self-mending talent. Without this ability, people would all end up in the scrap yard before they reached adulthood.

What enables the body to achieve such a feat is the immune system. One aspect of the immune system is to ward off germs, but it has another responsibility that is less glamorous but perhaps more important. Your child has an army of tens of thousands of microscopic cells that patrol the body constantly, ready to fight and do repairs when something goes wrong. The process of healing starts at the instant an injury occurs.

 Essential

Those emergency workers that have already arrived at the scene send out a signal to the rest of the body so that more help can be recruited. The sudden rush of cells and activity, in addition to the redirection of blood flow, causes the outward manifestation of swelling and redness around the cut skin.

When the skin is cut, pain and bleeding are the first things that a child experiences. On a microscopic level, the disrupted tissue and blood vessels immediately try to halt the blood loss by forming a crude barricade in the form of a soft scab. This barricade is relatively weak, but it can be erected extremely rapidly and forms an effective barrier to stop bleeding. At the same time, the body's immune cells rush to ground zero and set up a makeshift disaster zone so that rescue-worker cells can be flagged down and join the process of repair.

Regular traffic in the blood vessels surrounding the area of injury is temporarily redirected so that rescue workers can reach the disaster zone quickly. Pain is the alarm system the body uses to alert central command (the brain) that tissue damage has occurred. One of the brain's priorities is to pay attention to the area of injury and protect it from being further traumatized.

It Ain't Pretty

The process of repair and remodeling is a messy deal. In fact, tissue repair can be compared to a major home-improvement project. Imagine the state of your home while it is undergoing remodeling. With construction workers going in and out of your house, demolishing walls and generating tons of dust and debris in the process, the task of rebuilding isn't pretty. But it's a necessary chaos that the body must tolerate before the project is finished and your house is better than before.

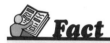 **Fact**

During the process of healing, a yellowish sticky substance may appear. This is called granulation tissue. This substance can look similar to pus, but there is usually less of it. It is the accumulation of the raw material the body is using to repair the damaged tissue, plus some repair cells. As long as there is no spreading redness or swelling, there is usually little cause for concern.

The same process goes on when the body is trying to repair that nasty gash on your child's knee. It's a necessary transition process, and the body is not going to look too pretty when it's doing its repairs. Swelling, redness, pain, and temporary restriction of movement are all part of the normal and expected inconvenience during tissue repair. Many parents interpret these outward signs as evidence of an impending infection, but these signs are often normal. The next section will explain the best way to differentiate signs of infection from the appearance of a healthy healing wound.

Infection Versus Healing

Distinguishing infection from normal healing isn't always an easy task. Sometimes even physicians can have a hard time differentiating between the two processes. However, there are some general guidelines to follow when making this decision.

Progression Is Paramount

One of the most helpful clues in distinguishing infection from healing is the way the appearance of the wound is changing. If redness is present, but its area of involvement and intensity is diminishing, this usually means that the wound is on its way to a smooth healing. On the other hand, if the redness spreads to a larger area and pain intensifies, the presence of infection becomes more likely.

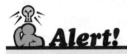

Alert!

At any time, if you are not sure whether the wound is looking better, do not hesitate to contact your doctor for an appointment. Sometimes it is very difficult to tell whether a wound is getting infected, and a doctor might consider performing additional laboratory tests to help make the distinction.

This is the rationale behind the practice some doctors use of taking a pen and drawing a line along the boundary of redness during the examination of a wound. This way, when the wound is checked again on the following day, it is easier to tell whether the area of redness is shrinking or growing.

Dirty Little Secret

The way the injury occurred is an important consideration when judging whether a wound is infected. For an injury that was incurred by a dirty object (such as a knee scraped on a sharp rock), physicians worry a lot more about the increased risk of infection than for a relatively clean wound (such as a cut from a brand-new razor). If the risk of bacterial contamination is high, some doctors elect to start the child on antibiotics even before signs of infection appear. This is especially true if the edge of the wound is jagged. A smooth and straight cut is a lot easier for the body to repair than a crooked cut.

Hydrogen Peroxide Abuse

Hydrogen peroxide has been touted as the miracle chemical of the century. Its uses include water purification, bleaching of commercial products, and use as a cleaning agent. However, when it comes to its medicinal uses, it has a long history of being abused and misused.

When you pour hydrogen peroxide onto wounded tissue, the wound immediately starts to bubble, a process that is followed by an intense pain. People used to think that this meant the antiseptic properties of hydrogen peroxide were kicking in. Scientists now know that this is actually an indication that healthy tissue is dying.

Collateral Damage

In fact, physicians of the past are part of the misconception problem. Decades ago, physicians were trained that the antiseptic quality of hydrogen peroxide was useful in cleaning open wounds and preventing wound infections. It is a common chemical found in most emergency departments. Recent studies, on the other hand, have shown that hydrogen peroxide actually impedes wound healing.

When hydrogen peroxide is applied to the wound, it combines with a natural chemical in human tissue. This combination generates oxygen and water. The concentrated amount of oxygen that is generated can kill off any bacteria that may be contaminating the wound, but it also kills healthy tissue in the body at the same time. The type of killing that is done by the concentrated oxygen is toxic to the human body. It kills anything alive indiscriminately, whether it's bacteria or healthy human cells. When the body is trying to repair the wound by sending in a microscopic repair crew, these cells can fall victim to the random killing by hydrogen peroxide.

To prevent wound infection, there are many more precise ways to kill the bacteria without hurting the healthy tissues in the body. Antibiotics are the best way to ward off infection, and they are more commonly used today than in the past.

Bring Out the Dead

Along with its role in infection prevention, hydrogen peroxide has historically been used to get rid of dead tissue in a bad open wound. This has also been proven ineffective, and the majority of medical professionals have halted this practice.

 Essential

Previously, there was similar concern about the use of iodine in wound cleansing and tissue damage. Extensive research in the 1990s showed that even though iodine compounds do not have the same deleterious effect on healing as hydrogen peroxide, they do not promote healing. In some cases, they can slightly hamper healing. The current recommendation is that they are safe for short-term wound care, but chronic application should be avoided.

Instead of using hydrogen peroxide, most doctors use a sterile salt water to clean the wound. This salt water is often drawn into a syringe and squirted into the wound to clean out any debris trapped inside the wound. Your child may need to be sedated or given pain medication prior to such treatment.

Ugly Scars

Formation of scar tissue is a common concern for parents, especially if the injury occurred at a conspicuous area of the body. There are many things that can be done to prevent scar formation. Most importantly, it is essential to prevention any infection of the wound. However, there are other factors that are completely beyond the control of doctors or parents when it comes to wound repair and scar formation. Genetics plays an important role.

To Sew or Not to Sew

Whether a skin laceration needs sewing, or stitches, is best determined by a trained medical professional. The circumstances of the injury, the location of the wound, and the age of your child are all important factors to be considered when making this decision. Even though most wounds heal without incident, the cosmetic result may be significantly better if a deep cut is sewn with sutures.

Generally speaking, a cut on the face or the hand needs special attention because scarring in these areas is undesirable and may interfere with bodily function. In addition, any injury involving open skin is at risk of getting infected. The doctor may need to clean the wound first before sewing it up. Some wounds are purposely left open (unstitched) because sewing up a badly contaminated wound can trap the bacteria inside, which can cause an even more serious deep tissue infection. When in doubt, it's wisest to have your child evaluated by a doctor. The doctor will make the ultimate decision about whether to suture the laceration or not.

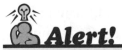

Alert!

Whenever the injury involves open skin, make sure that your child is not behind on his tetanus shot. A tetanus booster is recommended when your child turns eleven, and then every ten years after that. Contrary to popular belief, your child does not need to be punctured by a rusty nail in order to get tetanus. Any open wound is susceptible to the tetanus infection.

In the past ten years, the use of a superglue-like substance has become increasingly common in the treatment of minor skin cuts. Often known as Liquid Bandage, this can be the best choice of therapy for treating skin cuts in parts of the body that do not have a lot of forces pulling the skin apart. Most doctors are trained to use these adhesives, and they will offer this option when it's appropriate. If it is not offered, politely inquire about the possibility of using it. Your child's injury may not be a suitable candidate for this technique.

Keloid Scars
Some people are more prone to form large scar tissues even after a relatively minor skin injury. This tendency to form scars is largely a genetic trait. Keloid scars are much bulkier than normal scars because the scar tissue spreads to areas of the skin beyond that of the initial wound.

Keloid scars are notoriously difficult to treat. The involvement of a plastic surgeon is often necessary to manage a particular prominent keloid, and even then a satisfactory outcome cannot be guaranteed.

The best way to avoid keloid scars is to prevent any skin trauma in the first place. If many family members tend to form keloid scars, you should not allow your child to have elective piercing, including the ears. Notify your surgeon in advance if your child needs to go under the knife. There might be an alternative, less-invasive approach to the operation that can minimize the appearance of ugly scars.

When the Dog Bites

Children and pets cannot always coexist peacefully under one roof. After all, pets are animals, and you can never predict their behavior with complete certainty. Older pets can become jealous of the arrival of a new infant, and they can vie for attention from the parents. Injuries caused by pets are a common pediatric concern.

Dogs

A dog may be man's best friend, but sometimes even the best of friends can turn on you. Children are more likely to be the victim of dog attacks, not only because of their small size but also because they tend not to respect the personal space of pets. Frequently, dogs bite young children because they view them as competitors for food, especially when children play with their food bowls.

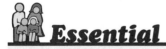 *Essential*

A common misconception is that human bites are a lot more dangerous than animal bites because the bacteria living in the human mouth are believed to be more vicious and virulent. Recent studies have shown that this is not the case. The chance of a wound infection is about equal for human bites and animal bites.

If the skin is broken from a dog bite, immediately clean the area well with soap and water to wash away any germs. If there is bleeding, the bite should be evaluated by a doctor. This is especially important if the bite occurred on the hand or the face. A doctor will often prescribe antibiotics for deep bite wounds to prevent infections and will check the date of the last tetanus vaccination.

If the bite is superficial and minor, all you need to do is apply topical antibiotics to the bite and allow the wound to heal on its own. If you see any of the signs of infection mentioned on page 150, seek medical attention immediately.

Cats

Cat bites are somewhat less common than dog bites, but when they occur, they are more dangerous. Cat bites are more likely to become infected for many reasons. For one, cats are carnivores. They have razor-sharp teeth that are more likely going to puncture and cut deeper than the omnivorous dentition of dogs. Furthermore, cats often harbor a specific type of bacteria in their mouths. This bacterium can cause an infection. Called cat-scratch disease, this can become a chronic infection that causes persistent fever, swollen glands, and headaches. This type of bacteria is more often found in the mouth of kittens than adult cats.

Rabies

Fortunately, rabies is a relatively rare condition in human beings. Otherwise, this deadly infection would be responsible for killing thousands of the people who are bitten by animals each year. In the United States, rabies is almost always caused by wild animals instead of domesticated ones. However, it is still prudent to check the rabies status of a dog if your child is bitten. Check with animal control if the status cannot be ascertained from the pet owner.

If your child is bitten by any type of wild animal, bring him to the emergency room immediately. Thorough cleaning of the bite wound is by far the most important step in preventing rabies. If the exact animal responsible for the biting can be identified and captured, it will be quarantined and evaluated for signs of rabies.

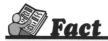 **Fact**

Contrary to what most people believe, most cases of rabies in the United States are not contracted from dogs. The animals that most commonly carry the rabies germ in this country are bats, raccoons, skunks, and coyotes. Even though squirrels do carry the virus, transmission from these small rodents is rare because they tend to die of the disease before they have a chance to bite anyone.

Turtles and Other Reptiles

Turtles can make good pets because they are relatively low maintenance and do not require a large living space to be content. Other reptiles, including snakes, iguanas, and lizards, can also be kept in small containers.

However, these reptiles can carry the salmonella bacteria. Hand-washing after handling these pets is a must to prevent contracting salmonellosis. If your child gets bitten by one of these animals, you should have him checked by the pediatrician if the skin is broken and there is bleeding. Even a small amount of bleeding can be a cause for concern. Once the skin barrier is breached, the salmonella bacteria can enter into the bloodstream. Salmonella is responsible for causing bloody diarrhea and a severe blood infection that can spread to the brain.

When the Bee Stings

As the weather gets warmer during the summer months, bugs thrive in the comfortable environment. Any outdoor activity is likely going to be plagued by swarms of bugs. At the same time, your children are likely to wear less due to the hot temperature, and as a consequence they literally become bug bait for these hungry little pests.

When Mosquitoes Attack

Mosquito bites are extremely common, and these little flying buggers seem to have a predilection for certain individuals' blood. You have probably noticed this in your family. Some people are plagued with bites, but others are mysteriously spared. Children are a prime target for mosquito bites because their bodies emit more heat. This is enough to attract mosquitoes, who then find that their tender skin is perfect for a good bite.

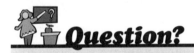

Question?

How can I tell if my child has chickenpox or mosquito bites?
Look carefully at the distribution of the rash on your child's body. Mosquito bites only occur on the exposed parts of the body. Therefore, they are very unusual on the upper thighs and buttocks. Fleabites tend to be focused on the lower legs, whereas chickenpox spots can occur anywhere on the body.

Most mosquito bites create nothing more than an annoying itch that can last more than two weeks. Some individuals develop localized allergic reaction to the bites, and the redness can persist for more than a month. The best way to alleviate the itching is to use a topical hydrocortisone cream, which is widely available over the counter. Avoid excessive scratching if possible. Breakage of the skin due to heavy scratching can lead to bacterial skin infection.

In 1999, when more cases of West Nile virus started appearing in North America, widespread panic swept through the nation. Parents prohibited their children from playing outdoors, and soccer games were canceled. It is now clear that children are at low risk for contracting the infection, and even if they are infected, they are unlikely going to suffer serious problems.

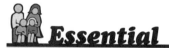

Essential

The rampant media coverage of the West Nile virus has blown this infection completely out of proportion. Out of 4,146 total reported cases of West Nile virus, there were 284 fatalities, but none of them was under the age of twelve. In the years since 1999, only one child under the age of eighteen has died from the West Nile virus.

If your mosquito-bitten child suffers from a persistent high fever that lasts longer than four days, and also has a stiff neck and confusion, seek medical attention immediately. In the unlikely event that he has swelling of the brain from the West Nile virus, aggressive medical intervention can generally help him recover successfully.

Flea Market

Fighting off a flea infestation can be one of the most aggravating experiences that any parents have to face. These annoying little pests are hard to kill, and they seem to have the ability to regenerate themselves out of nowhere. It's not uncommon to make three or four attempts to eradicate these bugs before you finally succeed, and at that point you would still be among the lucky ones.

Similar to mosquitoes, fleas have certain individual prefer-ence for their target. Some children are completely spared, yet others are eaten alive. This preference by fleas has nothing to do with blood types.

Fleas flourish during the warm summer months, and they become dormant during colder weather. When a flea problem arises in your household, there are several things you can do:

- If you have pets, call your veterinarian. Vets are gener-ally the most qualified experts to help you get through the problem.
- Treat your carpet and furniture with a flea powder or spray. Don't be cheap when shopping for a commercial powder.
- Prevent your children from playing on grass. Remember, fleas do not just live on pets. Most of them live in the soil and in the grass.

If your child has already been bitten by fleas, over-the-counter hydrocortisone creams are very effective in relieving the itch. Try to keep your child from scratching the fleabites. Bacterial skin infection is common from fleabites that are excessively scratched.

The Spider Strikes Back

Spider bites aren't nearly as common as people think. The reason is that spiders do not bite people because they are hun-gry. They bite because they fear for their lives. Imagine you are a little teeny spider and a creature more than a hundred times your size is about to squash you. Wouldn't you at least consider striking back in self-defense?

Because spiders bite for self-preservation and not for suste-nance, there usually is a single bite mark on the skin. They usu-ally just bite you and try to quickly scurry away to safety. They do not stay around and bite you over and over again.

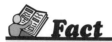 *Fact*

Even though most people are deathly afraid of the black widow spider, these small creatures are actually not as poisonous as people think. For adults, they never cause any fatality. In children, they rarely cause life-threatening problems, but they can cause intense pain and muscle cramps.

The brown recluse spider is responsible for most of the serious spider bites in children. This spider has a relatively large body, and it likes to hide in dark and damp areas in the yard. Once threatened, it will strike back by biting. The bite wound is intensely painful at first, but gradually it becomes itchy and forms a blister. The blister may rupture and the area around the blister turn deep red. It can take up to a few weeks before the bite resolves completely.

If you believe your child has been bitten by a spider, talk to a medical professional on the phone before rushing to the office. The doctor or nurse will ask you a series of questions to identify the source of the bite. If a spider bite is likely, your doctor may want to examine your child directly.

Stung by a Bee

Usually, a bee sting is not a big deal unless the victim develops an allergic reaction to the bee venom. If the latter is the case, a small sting can trigger a life-threatening emergency.

Since you don't know whether your child is allergic to bee stings until the first time she is stung, it pays to be vigilant when your child is playing in an outdoor area where bees are common. If you notice a sting that is followed by facial or lip swelling and drooling, do not hesitate to call for emergency assistance. Every second counts during a whole-body allergic reaction.

If your child has already had an experience with severe allergic reaction due to insect stings, you should always carry injectable adrenaline with you whenever your child is playing outside. If you witness facial swelling or breathing difficulty after a sting, immediately inject the adrenaline according to your pediatrician's instructions. This could be a life-saving maneuver.

CHAPTER 12

Childhood Obesity

C hildhood obesity is on the rise, and public awareness of this epidemic is increasing as well, thanks to the constant media barrage of news stories and reports. Simply walk down the street and you'll likely encounter many children (and adults) who clearly carry more weight than what is healthy for them. Some people perceive being overweight as only a cosmetic issue. Obesity is the major risk factor for diabetes in children, and diabetes not only shortens life, but it greatly diminishes the quality of life as well.

Definition of Childhood Obesity

The very definition of obesity is controversial. Some people measure it by using a standard growth chart to compare a child with other children of the same age. Others use a ratio of the body weight and the height of the child. In addition, there are more sophisticated methods of measuring the percentage of body fat. The bottom line is that there is no single guideline that can determine whether a child's weight is healthy. Multiple factors must be considered simultaneously to determine the ideal weight for your child.

The Fallacy of the Growth Chart

Using weight alone as a criterion to decide whether someone is overweight is clearly flawed.

Many people focus too much on weight and neglect to consider other factors that determine whether someone is healthy. It's misleading to use weight as the only criterion for judging your child's health.

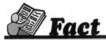 **Fact**

Overweight children tend to be taller than average because the additional fat tissue makes more growth hormones to stimulate vertical growth. However, this early growth spurt does not translate into taller adult height.

It is also dangerous to use the absolute weight to figure out how much overweight your child is compared to the average. Using this weight difference is a bad idea for many reasons. First of all, your child may be heavier because she is taller, and it would not be a good idea for her to weigh the same as someone of average height. Secondly, it is unhealthy and dangerous for a growing child to lose weight to match an ideal body weight. A child's body is genetically programmed to grow and gain weight. Going against this tendency is detrimental to the health.

If a child is determined to be unhealthily overweight, the best thing to do is to maintain the current weight as much as possible and have her grow into her weight. As she grows taller, she will naturally attain her ideal body weight.

The Body Mass Index
The body mass index (BMI) is one of the most helpful tools for screening children for being overweight, but it's by no means perfect. Used incorrectly, it can be misinterpreted and abused. After determining your child's BMI, it must be interpreted by a physician or dietician according to your child's age and overall

health condition. Two children with the exact same BMI can have different risks of being overweight because their age and growth stage are different.

BMI can be misleading in many circumstances. For example, a professional shot-putter or boxer typically has a BMI that is much higher than the standard threshold for obesity. However, common sense can tell you that these athletes are more than fit. What skews the index is the above-average lean body mass in these individuals.

The BMI alone is insufficient to paint an accurate picture of the overall health status for a child. When it comes to determining your child's healthy weight, pediatricians factor many things into consideration, including the age of the child, past medical history, current nutritional status, height and lean body mass, and other medical conditions that might influence weight. It is no simple matter. If you have any concern about your child's weight, bring it to the attention of your pediatrician or a dietician. Either of these health professionals will be glad to evaluate your child and address your questions.

Baby Fat

Many parents believe it is okay for toddlers to be chubby. The term "baby fat" is often used to justify an overweight child. The complacency that comes with this type of thinking is dangerous. If your child is older than eighteen months and his weight is significantly high relative to his height, your child may be at risk for becoming an overweight adult. If you are unsure about whether the weight is excessive, talk to your pediatrician. While it is important to monitor your child's weight, you have to make the distinction between a chubby child and a chubby baby. The age of the child is paramount when it comes to evaluating obesity.

If your toddler is over the age of eighteen months and appears overweight to you, do not dismiss it by thinking that it's just baby fat. Ask your pediatrician to evaluate your child to make sure that he is not overweight and unhealthy. Do it as soon as possible before the problem becomes a bigger one.

Essential

Children learn by example. They develop their eating habits by observing the adults around them. Make sure you set a good example for your child by choosing healthy snacks and consuming lots of fresh fruits and vegetables. Do not show open distaste for new or healthy foods. Your child will copy your reaction and become a picky eater.

The Worst Offenders

Soft-drink companies and distributors of snack chips may not appear sinister, but they are partially to blame for the epidemic of obesity in developed countries. While myriad other factors may contribute to the overall deterioration of children's health, the increase in the consumption of soft drinks by children is perhaps the single most important reason why childhood obesity is on the rise.

If parents and children can change just one thing about their diet, they need to curtail the consumption of soft drinks. Making this single change can result in a great reduction in total caloric intake, and the impact on health is immeasurable.

Sweet Drinks

Unfortunately, through decades of successful marketing, sports drinks like Gatorade and Powerade have made tremendous strides in making the public think that they are good for the body. Advertisements and television commercials always pair these drinks with elite athletes and great-looking bodies. The aim is to give the impression that by drinking these things, the consumer will become strong and energetic like these athletes.

Unfortunately, producers of these drinks have done a brilliant job with this marketing strategy, which has been hugely successful. Very few consumers think these drinks are unhealthful.

But sports drinks are packed with sugar. They are not as bad as soft drinks, but they're still a far cry from being good for the body. It sounds reasonable that the body needs to be replenished with salts and sugar after strenuous activities. But unless the athlete has just finished a marathon or the Tour de France, these drinks replenish much more sugar than the body needs, and certainly more sugars than salts. For casual weekend warriors and young athletes, fluid replacement is more important than anything else. The best way to rehydrate the body is with plain water. The calories burned off during exercise will be resupplied with the next meal. It isn't necessary to get the sugar from these drinks.

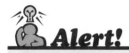

Alert!

Natural 100-percent fruit juices have just as many calories, if not more, than nondiet soft drinks. A twelve-ounce bottle of grape soda has 159 calories. The same amount of natural grape juice contains 228 calories. This shocking truth tells the danger of consuming large quantities of fruit juices, even those without any added sugar. It is much healthier to eat fresh fruit than to drink fresh fruit juice.

The powerful juice industry isn't far behind the sports-drink manufacturers on their quest to brainwash the public. It is easy to think that 100-percent natural juices are good, if not essential, as part of a healthful diet. One of the most frequent questions parents ask their pediatricians is when they should introduce juice to their babies. Most doctors and dieticians agree that infants should stay on milk and water for as long as possible. Juice isn't necessary at all. Older children should limit their juice intake.

Fruit juice should be an occasional treat for children, as its high sugar content means it is basically a liquid form of dessert.

Recently, a team of Massachusetts scientists conducted research involving 100 volunteer adolescents. They monitored the consumption of sugary drinks for these teens for six months. Half of them were constantly encouraged to cut down on their intake of sweet drinks, while the other half continued to drink to their hearts' content.

At the end of six months, those who tried to limit their sweet drinks were successful in doing so 82 percent of the time, and they lost a modest amount of weight. On the other hand, the group that continued to drink sugary fluids gained weight. These children didn't change any other aspects of their diet besides the sweet drinks, but this single change was sufficient to make a difference in weight in as little as six months.

What can you do if your child cannot drink soft drinks, sports drinks, or even natural fruit juices? Not having all these other options actually makes it simpler. Just remember "water and milk." It has been shown that low-fat milk consumption actually helps some people lose weight. Of course, water has no calories, so it's fine to drink at any time. You can't go wrong with sticking to water and milk. You will also be amazed at how much this helps limit your calorie intake.

The Chip on Your Shoulder

Potato chips and other crunchy snacks have made tremendous inroads into the lives of millions of children. A recent news story illustrates just how entrenched these snacks have become in the lives of schoolchildren. One school's attempt to ban "hot" Cheetos from campus resulted in a full-scale revolt by the pupils. Many of them could not imagine a life without these spicy snacks. Their popularity demonstrates not only the manufacturer's success in marketing their product but the role these snacks play in the rising tide of childhood obesity.

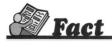 **Fact**

Due to the health risk posed by trans-fatty acids, in 2003 the U.S. Food and Drug Administration (FDA) required all food manufacturers to label the amount of trans-fatty acids in packaged foods. By January 2006, all food-processing companies must comply with this regulation. As a result of this new mandate, many companies have reduced or completely eliminated the use of trans-fat in their products.

These snacks, including potato chips, cheese curls, pork rinds, tortilla chips, and pretzels, have no real nutritional value. Beyond the excess of carbohydrate they deliver, they are often fried in oil composed of infamous trans-fatty acids. Trans-fatty acids are naturally present in small amounts in animal fat. The snack industry has artificially converted vegetable oil into this type of fat because it tastes good and is much easier to preserve. Trans-fatty acids have absolutely no nutritional benefit to the human body, and their presence undeniably increases cholesterol levels. The combination of empty carbohydrate calories and trans-fat makes these chips completely devoid of any redeeming value. They are as unhealthful as anything could get.

Snack Habits

It is inevitable that children will feel hungry between meals, and these are the times when they are most tempted to snack on junk foods. There is nothing wrong with snacking itself, but parents have to be especially vigilant when it comes to children's snacks.

Unfortunately, the grocery-store aisles are stocked with an abundance of processed foods and sugary snacks. With colorful packaging that often incorporates popular cartoon characters, food companies are extremely adept at direct marketing to the young consumer. Some of these snacks advertise that they are loaded with essential vitamins and nutrients, but they typically contain an excessive amount of calories and sugar. It is much better to acquire the vitamins from fresh fruits and vegetables. It is not necessary to eat these sweet snacks to get enough vitamins for the body.

The best advice is to keep a big fruit bowl always available in the kitchen. This way, when your child gets hungry, she will not be rummaging through the cupboard looking for cookies or chips. Children often come home from school feeling famished. If a good selection of healthy snacks isn't readily available, they will end up eating high-calorie snacks.

Childhood Diabetes

Diabetes has become a scourge of epidemic proportion in recent decades. Most pediatric health experts agree that the primary culprit is the rise in childhood obesity. Not only does this condition doom the child to a lifetime of constant blood tests and medications, it wreaks havoc on the body, taking a toll that causes it to deteriorate and ultimately leads to an early grave.

Regardless of the type, diabetes is a condition in which the body loses its natural ability to regulate and utilize blood sugar. As a result, blood-sugar levels fluctuate wildly in children with diabetes. The bloodstream gets inundated with sugar right after a meal, and this abnormally high level of sugar causes chemical changes in the blood vessels. These chemical alterations do not cause symptoms early on, but the cumulative effects of these changes are devastating in the long run.

Insulin is the hormone that triggers blood sugar in the bloodstream to be transported to the body's cells so the sugar can be utilized as an energy source for the body's functions. In diabetics, there is either a deficiency of insulin or the cells in the body stop responding to the signal conveyed by existing insulin.

Type 1 Diabetes

Type 1 diabetes used to be called juvenile type diabetes, but that has become a misnomer now that more children are diagnosed with type 2 diabetes than type 1. Before the dramatic increase in childhood obesity, children rarely got type 2 diabetes. The rampant overweight problem in children quickly changed all that.

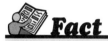 **Fact**

Type 1 diabetes is hypothesized to originate from an immunologic attack within one's own body on the organ that produces insulin. Without an adequate amount of insulin, the body cannot transport the sugar from the bloodstream into the cells. Therefore, the sugar in the blood remains abnormally high, while the cells in the body starve.

Symptoms start relatively quickly when children first come down with type 1 diabetes. These include increased thirst, urination, and weight loss, despite a ravenous appetite. If undiagnosed, the weight loss can be quite drastic. Lack of energy and vomiting are warning signs that the diabetes is far out of control. Unless these children seek medical help urgently, they may drift into a coma.

Type 2 Diabetes

Type 2 diabetes is primarily the result of being overweight. As obesity sets in, the body's natural hormone-control mechanism fails, and the cells stop responding to the signals from insulin. Consequently, the insulin level in type 2 diabetics is initially elevated to compensate for the lack of response. Eventually, the body's insulin production shuts down after working excessively for an extended period of time.

Symptoms associated with type 2 diabetes generally occur more insidiously than with type 1 diabetes. The body initially tries to compensate for the insulin insensitivity, but after working overtime for so long, it ultimately fails. Symptoms are similar to those associated with type 1 diabetes except that they are less acute and less pronounced. Frequent yeast infections and slow wound-healing can be early signs of the illness. Children with type 2 diabetes are less likely to develop coma from the onset of diabetes because the symptoms tend to appear gradually.

Type 1.5 Diabetes

Some children with diabetes have elements of both type 1 and type 2 diabetes. Pediatric endocrinologists (specialists who take care of children with diabetes) have termed this condition "type 1.5 diabetes."

The initial symptoms for these children consist of a hybrid between type 1 and type 2 diabetes. In particular, these children tend to be more overweight than children with type 1 diabetes.

Establishing the Diagnosis

Early signs of type 2 diabetes include rapid weight gain and the appearance of dark pigmentation around the neck and the armpits. These are ominous findings, but they do not always precede type 2 diabetes. Clinicians usually order screening tests for diabetes if these physical findings are present in a patient.

Laboratory evaluation typically involves a blood sugar level, a urine test for excessive sugar leaking into the urine, other hormone levels (including thyroid hormone), and a cholesterol level. Fortunately, confirming the diagnosis for diabetes is relatively straightforward. It's what comes after the diagnosis that is complicated.

Complications of Diabetes

There are too many potential complications from diabetes to be listed here. The most devastating include blindness, amputation of the feet, heart attacks, and strokes.

All of the horrific conditions listed above result from damage within the blood vessels due to an elevated blood sugar level. Diabetes is the leading cause of blindness in the United States, and it is also the leading cause of amputation. It also contributes to the high death rate from cardiovascular diseases, such as heart attacks and strokes.

The damage to these organs starts immediately when diabetes first sets in, regardless of the age of the child. The sooner the blood sugar is brought under control, the more you can minimize the long-term disability caused by diabetes. Frequent evaluation by an eye doctor is absolutely essential for children with diabetes.

Management

Once diabetes strikes, there is no cure for it. Consequently, it's paramount to regulate blood sugar to minimize the damage that diabetes can do to the body. Most children rely on insulin injections to control their blood sugar, but a very small minority can be managed with oral medications. Regardless of the insulin regimen, healthy nutrition and a regular exercise program are the most important components of any diabetic management plan. A lifestyle change is often necessary for these patients, especially for those with type 2 diabetes.

Insulin can be a particularly dangerous medication. If it is given inappropriately (at the wrong time or in the wrong dosage), it can quickly kill a child. Even if the correct dose is given at the right time, if the child already has low blood sugar for whatever reason (such as a missed dinner or sleeping in), the usual dose of insulin can lower the blood sugar to a life-threatening level.

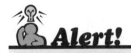

Alert!

It's a tricky business getting children to stick to their insulin regimen, which requires them to measure their blood sugar levels meticulously and consistently. For a child who is not yet mature enough to manage her own insulin injections, the parents or caregiver must step in to supervise her care.

At the same time, studies show that a very aggressive insulin regimen—one that lowers blood sugar more than the traditional approach—can prevent or delay long-term complications from diabetes. So a regimen that is too lax is less risky in the here and now, but the regimented child suffers permanent organ damage in the long run. A more strict insulin regimen has higher risk of causing dangerously low blood sugars, but it protects the patient from permanent disability. It's a fine line between balancing the risk of management and long-term disability.

The Danger of Dieting

Many people perceive dieting as a periodic event. When a person's body weight becomes excessive, he might decide it's time to cut down the food intake until his weight drops. Once the weight returns to an acceptable level, it's okay to eat more again. This is the classic roller-coaster diet, and this way of eating and living is not only harmful, but also unpleasant. Dieters feel that there is a constant struggle with their weight. When a parent imposes this kind of thinking upon a child, the regimen can strain the parent-child relationship and make the child feel helpless. This type of eating pattern should never happen. If it is already happening, this cycle must be broken.

Going on a Diet

First of all, it's not lack of will power that leads to obesity or over-eating. More often, obesity is caused by an eating habit picked up over the years from family or friends. Clearly, no one ever intends to become overweight. Regardless, changing one's eating habits is challenging.

One of the biggest myths about achieving an ideal weight is that overweight children must go on a diet to lose weight. This is perhaps the single worst misconception in the world of nutrition. In fact, if done inappropriately, it is dangerous and potentially life threatening.

Unlike adults, the bodies of young children are designed to grow, which means that they need to gain weight. The genetic blueprint of a growing child instructs the body to grow taller and bigger, and weight gain is virtually inevitable. Opposing this natural tendency is not only difficult, it can be hazardous to a child's health.

 Essential

The notion of "going on a diet" reinforces the idea that eating healthily is only done periodically, and only once someone becomes overweight. Every child should eat healthily, and it should be done throughout a child's life. Even for skinny people, frequent consumption of junk food and sweet snacks is bad for their health, and this practice should never be condoned.

What can you do to help an obese child attain a healthy weight? Since children do grow, you can use this to your advantage. As they grow taller, if they're able to maintain the same weight or just gain a small amount of weight, these children will eventually grow into their height. If they are able to accomplish this weight maintenance, there is a good chance that they can achieve a healthy weight as an adult.

The Low-Carb Craze

The media in the past decade have blitzed the public with miraculous success stories about individuals losing an astonishing amount of weight by following a diet that is low in carbohydrates. Many parents have experienced some success themselves, and they are eager to apply the same regimen to their children. However, it is unclear whether this type of extremely strict diet is safe for children.

Carbohydrates are converted to sugar once they get into the body. The human brain can use only one type of fuel—sugar. If the body is starved of this vital nutrient, the brain essentially goes into an emergency mode. It does not function well when the brain is desperately trying to budget its sole source of energy. This constant state of starvation certainly doesn't bode well for the development of the brain in the long run.

The general consensus of pediatricians is that a restrictive low-carbohydrate diet is not recommended for children. It is more important to eat a well-balanced diet.

Going Overboard

Children who are overweight are especially at risk of developing an eating disorder. After years of obsession about weight control, many children become stringent in their eating and food selection. Some of them become bulimics who spiral down into a cycle of binging and purging.

In addition, make sure you have some flexibility in controlling your child's dietary intake. Prohibiting your child from enjoying a piece of the birthday cake on her own birthday is just plain unreasonable. A single indulgence on a rare occasion is not going to break her healthy eating habit. Going overboard and having absolutely no wiggle room can possibly encourage your child to rebel and start hoarding sweets secretly.

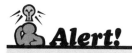
Alert!

Many children who suffer from eating disorders either are overweight or were once overweight. The most important message for children who are overweight is that they should not refrain from eating. Instead, they must make smart choices when it comes to *what* they are eating.

Smart Food Choices

A healthy diet does not mean eating very little or limiting one's choice of food to just lettuce and carrots. A healthy diet consists of a balance of fruits and vegetables, lean meat, and a good portion of dairy products. At the same time, it strictly limits the consumption of sweet snacks. Most importantly, it means never being hungry.

One of the worst things a child can do is to skip breakfast. Doing so sabotages any hopes of a healthy meal plan for the remainder of the day. Skipping breakfast invariably makes the child famished before lunch. This extreme hunger can cloud the judgment and prevent the child from making good decisions when it comes to snacking or picking out healthful food from the lunch menu.

The Fat Paranoia

Fat has been the scapegoat for the obesity epidemic for many decades. It has gotten a worse rap than it deserves. The truth is that fat is an essential part of a good diet. Without it, human beings cannot survive. The human brain is composed mostly of fat. During the stage of rapid brain development in childhood, fat is essential for the growth of a healthy mind.

The higher requirement for fat during the toddler years, when brain development is rapid, is the reason pediatricians and dieticians recommend providing whole milk to children until they are two years old. Low-fat and nonfat (or skim) milk may not supply an adequate amount of fat to a growing brain.

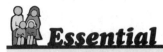

Essential

To make things easier, always keep a bowl of fresh fruit on the kitchen table. When your kids come back from school, they won't have to rummage through the cabinet looking for some junk food. They can snack on an apple or banana instead.

This is not to say that children should consume an unlimited amount of fat. The body derives more calories from fat than from an equal portion of other types of food. Make sure your child's diet is balanced, which means it should include vegetables, fruits, meats, dairy products, and grains.

The Cholesterol Controversy

Just like fat, cholesterol has gotten its share of unfair negative publicity. Its role in heart disease and stroke is undeniable, but it's not always true that a diet low in cholesterol will guarantee you a low cholesterol level in the blood.

Cholesterol is a type of fat found only in animal tissue. It is especially abundant in organ meat and certain types of seafood. A strict vegetarian who avoids all meat, dairy products, and eggs would not derive any cholesterol from the diet. However, these vegetarians could still have dangerously high cholesterol levels in the body. The reason for this is that the human body generates its own cholesterol.

Many people are unaware that cholesterol is also an essential component of the body. It is the material from which many human hormones are derived. In addition, its role inside the brain is indispensable. Without cholesterol, no human being could survive. That is the reason the body generates its own cholesterol, even if none is ingested from any food matter.

It is still a good idea to avoid taking in excessive cholesterol in the diet. The body generates the majority of its cholesterol, and a diet rich in cholesterol will elevate the blood level of cholesterol even more. However, cholesterol avoidance can be taken to the extreme. Some parents are so afraid of cholesterol that they eliminate all foods high in cholesterol from their children's diet. This is generally not a good thing for the following reasons.

Many nutritious foods that are high in cholesterol are also rich sources of vitamins and protein. Eggs and liver are great examples of these types of food. In the process of completely eliminating them from the diet, parents also effectively take away many food choices from their children's menu. This is unnecessary and sends the wrong message to children about eating a balanced diet.

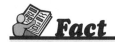 **Fact**

Foods that are high in cholesterol include most animal fat, organ meat, and dairy products. Lean meats have significantly less cholesterol than fat-laden meats. Low-fat dairy products are recommended for anyone older than two years of age.

Instead, it is recommended for children to eat a variety of foods, including some that may have cholesterol. As long as it is done in moderation, there is no reason to worry about raising cholesterol levels. For example, enjoying one egg a day does not pose any health risk as far as cholesterol is concerned. Occasional organ meat in the diet is also safe. Liver is an excellent source of vitamin B12, which is an essential vitamin for blood and brain development.

Moderation Is Healthy

Finally, listen to your child. When he says he's had enough, do not force him to finish the his food or clean his plate. If the leftover portion is excessive, save it for later or discard it. No one wants to advocate wasting food, so it's a better idea to serve less food next time if your child consistently cannot finish his meals. Forcing your child to eat everything on his plate when he is obviously full teaches him to ignore his internal satiety cues. This can easily lead to overeating in adulthood.

A Healthy Lifestyle

There is no short-term solution to achieving a healthy body weight, which is really a long-term pursuit. It requires a complete overhaul in lifestyle, including dietary and activity modifications. There are many wrong ways of doing things, and that's why it's particularly important to follow the advice of physicians and dieticians in guiding your child to the healthy goal.

Let's Get Moving

Today's children lead an increasingly sedentary lifestyle, just like their adult counterparts. To reverse this trend, it is paramount to first eliminate the indoor pastimes that suck up most of their time. Limiting television time goes a long way to this end. Pediatricians recommend that children watch no more than one hour of television a day. Parents can allow the child to select one or two programs that they want to watch, but they must stick to that schedule. When the program is over, the television goes off.

While video games are not intrinsically bad, it is important to limit the amount of time children spend playing them. Even with some of the more interactive titles, where children dance around on an electronic sensor pad on the floor, activity level is severely restricted. Time spent interacting with the video screen could be better spent engaging in outdoor activities.

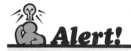

Alert!

Pediatricians recommend against using the television as a babysitter. It is enticing and extremely convenient, but it sets a bad precedent for the child to sit in front of the tube for extended periods of time. Furthermore, do not leave the television on during mealtimes. It encourages indiscriminate watching.

It's a Family Affair

By eating together healthily, the members of a family send and support the strong message that being healthy is a universal responsibility.

Families should have predictable mealtimes, when everyone sits down and has a healthy meal together. Eating a meal together at least once a day is extremely important to establish a healthy eating pattern for children. This ritual alone cuts down the consumption of potentially bad snacks with poor nutritional value. The mealtime should be a pleasant bonding experience, giving everyone a chance to relax and socialize.

Essential

A healthy family menu starts at the shopping stage. If you don't buy unhealthy snacks and soft drinks, you effectively remove the temptation to consume them. All members of the family must adhere to a strict shopping guideline. It does not work if the parent is a responsible shopper but the grandparents go out and buy junk foods.

In addition, families should schedule regular physical activities. Instead of sitting together on the living room couch and watching television, the entire family can go out for a walk or ride bikes together after dinner. It is much more difficult to exercise alone than to do it in the company of the people you love. Everyone can benefit from the extra physical exercise, regardless of health status. Remember, exercise doesn't have to be an unrelenting "death march." Make it into a game and incorporate fun elements into the activities.

Setting Realistic Goals

Even with the strategies mentioned above, it is always important to set realistic goals when it comes to lifestyle changes. Planning to go from a couch potato to running a marathon in less than four months is simply a setup for failure. Likewise, planning to switch from an unhealthy diet to a diet consisting of carrot sticks is equally impractical. The road to success is all about taking small steps and making the trek patiently. Old habits die hard. You can't expect to become healthy overnight.

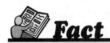 *Fact*

It is usually wise to change one thing at a time when it comes to food selection changes. The best idea is to cut out the worst offenders and then work your way down the list one by one. Soft drinks should go first, followed by other food items, such as crunchy snacks.

Before signing your child up for the soccer team, it's a good idea to improve her physical conditioning and stamina. It would be unfair to make her struggle on a team full of children who have been accustomed to running hours at a stretch. Start by taking an after-dinner stroll with your child, and gradually work it up to a brisk walk. Running a long distance (more than two miles) should be a distant goal, especially if you and your child are not used to running. It takes time and patience to see the result of regular exercise, but it's well worth the effort.

CHAPTER 13

Mental Health

A ll parents want to provide a nurturing environment so that their children can achieve their potential. Occasionally, despite the best intentions and effort, a child falls short of that goal because of other factors. One of the most common reasons that some children underachieve is attention deficit hyperactivity disorder (ADHD). Beyond ADHD, the increasing incidence of autism has made parents more aware and fearful of mental-health and behavioral issues. In addition, the impact of depression and anxiety disorders on children's lives has not always been recognized.

What Is ADHD?

ADHD is an official diagnosis in the manual of the American Psychiatric Association. It has strict criteria for its diagnosis, and there are objective ways for evaluating it. You might hear the terms attention deficit disorder (ADD) and ADHD used almost interchangeably in many references. There are some technical differences between children with ADD and ADHD, but for the purpose of this discussion, we'll focus on ADHD. Most of the discussion applies equally well to either condition, and the treatments of ADD and ADHD are identical.

The difference between ADD and ADHD is rather minor. Children with ADD lack the outward hyperactivity aspect of the disorder, even though their mind is racing. Frequently, these children are diagnosed later because they are not disruptive in class and they do not call attention to their lack of focus.

 Essential

If your child is performing poorly in school, ADHD should be in the back of your mind. No one, however, should jump to conclusions and automatically diagnose a child with ADHD with only a cursory understanding of the child's behavior. Remember, ADHD is a medical condition that can only be diagnosed by a medical professional.

Children with ADHD have a hard time controlling their thoughts and actions. They find it difficult to focus their attention on what they are doing, and they are easily distracted by irrelevant stimuli. While most young children have a shorter attention span than adults, children with ADHD generally have more problems focusing than other children of the same age.

A Common Diagnosis

According to the present medical database, about 8 percent of children in the United States are diagnosed with ADHD. That statistic translates into 4.5 million children. You may argue that the number is higher or lower, but you must admit there is no way to avoid this common issue.

The increasing prevalence of ADHD is probably due to a wider public awareness of the condition. It is unlikely that there are actually more children developing the condition than before. Instead, vigilant teachers, parents, and doctors are helping affected children to be appropriately diagnosed and treated.

Signs to Look For

What do you look for in your child if you suspect that he or she might have ADHD? Children with ADHD are often described as if they are being driven by a motor. The incessant activities usually do not involve the completion of any one task. Instead, they jump from one thing to the next, usually before finishing the tasks they have already started.

They also have a hard time paying attention to instructions. Frequently, they either fail to hear what you are saying to them or completely forget what you told them. Even though these children may actually have excellent memories, they often appear forgetful. It's their disorganization that prevents them from registering information.

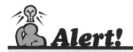

Alert!

As social awareness of this disorder grows, some children are being diagnosed with ADHD at an extremely young age. Even though children may show signs of ADHD before the age of six, it is virtually impossible to make a diagnosis before school age. If a health professional made an ADHD diagnosis before your child reached age six, you should consider consulting a child psychiatrist.

Almost all children behave in ways that fit these descriptions at one time or another, and these findings tend to wane with age. By the time most children are ready to enter school, they do not always behave impulsively, and their attention span is long enough for them to digest a short lesson. For children with ADHD, on the other hand, the traits that constitute this disorder seem to affect them much more often and with greater intensity than their peers.

If you suspect your child might have ADHD, bring up your concern with your pediatrician. A formal evaluation by the pediatrician or a pediatric psychiatrist is necessary to diagnose your child with ADHD. Typically, this means you will go through several question-and-answer sessions. The doctor may also collect written questionnaires from your child's teachers. There is no blood test, brain scan, or any other physical test that can aid in the diagnosis of ADHD.

Causes of ADHD

ADHD has a strong genetic basis. Children with ADHD are likely to have other family members with the condition. You should not feel guilty if you have passed on the ADHD trait to your child, just as you shouldn't feel guilty if you passed on the gene for curly hair. It's not really up to you to decide what genetic inheritance you give your children. Perhaps the ADHD trait will actually turn out to be a gift that your child can take advantage of, once the condition is under control.

The Sugar High

You have probably heard parents blaming candy bars and sweetened drinks for their children's rowdy behavior. Despite the popularity of this myth, there is absolutely no scientific evidence backing it. Scientists and pediatricians know that there is no such thing as a "sugar high," and the observation by many parents that their children tend to run around like wild beasts after a hit of sugar is purely anecdotal.

Video Games

Many parents are quick to blame the popularity of video games for the rise in past decades of ADHD. Despite the rapidly growing popularity of video games, however, the number of children diagnosed with ADHD has only risen gradually. If gaming were to blame for ADHD, then over half of the children in this country would have been diagnosed with ADHD already.

In fact, children with ADHD often excel at video games. Even though this is a common observation in children with ADHD, the explanation for this apparent paradox is hard to come by. While these children find it difficult to finish other tasks, they can remain intensely focused on a game for many hours. The child's ability to focus for an extended period of time on a video game leads some parents to believe that their child could not have ADHD.

Treatment Options

Pediatricians have developed vast clinical experience over the past few decades in treating children with ADHD. Sadly, too many children remain undiagnosed and do not get the help they need to overcome their attention problem. There are many options for parents to consider when treating their children for ADHD, but the most important is to bring the child's behavior to the attention of their pediatrician.

Consequences of Delaying Treatment

Parents might be reluctant to have their child labeled and treated, but the consequences of not dealing with the situation can be devastating. Without formal diagnosis and treatment for ADHD, children with this condition are likely to suffer through years of poor academic achievement and delinquency. Not only are they deprived of the opportunity to acquire the knowledge they need to succeed as an adult, the toll on their self-esteem is often irreparable. If intervention is introduced too late, the child will not benefit much from the belated treatment because they no longer believe in their innate ability and talent. More often than not, they end up scraping by through life as under-achieving adults.

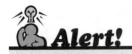
Alert!

If your child has an attention problem, it must be dealt with aggressively and early. Something must be done before his exuberance for learning and self-confidence start to flag from repeated failures. If your child truly has ADHD and is struggling in school, it would be extremely unfair to withhold valuable treatment options from him and prevent him from expressing his true talents.

Structure and Lists

Establishing a structured routine in your child's life is paramount; this is even more important if your child has ADHD. Because children with ADHD are more forgetful, having a daily schedule for the child to follow is a powerful way to help them organize their activities.

In addition, keeping lists as reminders can help your child stay on task and finish the tasks. This is a common technique used by adults with ADHD to keep their lives in order. Just make sure that the lists are kept in specific locations so that they are not misplaced.

Having another person who reminds them of things can be useful as well, but this is not always feasible. While parents can oversee their child's progress in school and remind them to finish their homework, this kind of assistance is not workable once the child is old enough to live independently. It is a good idea to gradually wean your child from your constant reminders before she enters young adulthood.

Medications

This is a dreaded option for many parents because they think placing their children on medication is tantamount to drugging them into passivity. Nothing could be further from the truth. Medications designed for ADHD are technically stimulants, but they have no stimulating effect on children with ADHD. Quite the opposite, these medications allow children to focus their attention more easily and to curb their hyperactivity. While the overall effect is that your child appears calmer, these medications do not have any sedating effect at all.

 Essential

Medications prescribed for ADHD allow your child to function the way he has always been meant to, without the disrupting influence of ADHD. If you think your child is behaving strangely on the medication, you could be seeing a side effect or another factor. Contact your doctor immediately if you have any concerns.

One of the most important aspects of ADHD treatment is close monitoring and regular follow-up exams. The first medication that the doctor prescribes for your child might not be the best. Furthermore, instead of being based on the child's weight, dosage is subjective and varies from child to child. The key in monitoring treatment is to continuallygauge the child's behavior and school performance on the medication. Carefully checking for potential side effects is equally important. It may take up to six months to determine the right medication at the appropriate dosage. Be patient, and understand that the process can be frustrating.

Dealing with Side Effects

The most common side effects associated with the stimulants that treat ADHD include loss of appetite, insomnia, vague stomach discomfort, and headaches. These side effects all typically lessen in intensity with time, once the body adapts to the medication. If a side effect becomes intolerable, your doctor will either reduce the dosage or switch to an alternative medication.

Follow-up exams are generally scheduled monthly. The physician monitors the child's weight and blood pressure at each visit. Inquiries into academic performance and sleep are routine. If a child is overmedicated, school performance may actually deteriorate rather than improve. Once again, the importance of monitoring your child closely while she is on the medication cannot be overemphasized. You should notify your doctor immediately if anything worries or alarms you.

Fear of Misdiagnosis

Since ADHD cannot be diagnosed with blood tests or brain scans, many parents are uncomfortable with the diagnosis and question its validity. This is a perfectly valid concern. You wouldn't want your child to take a medication that alters brain function for the wrong reason.

Since all children diagnosed and treated for ADHD require close monitoring and regular follow-up visits, your physician will notice if any prescribed medications are not working as intended or expected. The next step would be to investigate other possible causes of poor school performance. At the same time, it is important to remember that many children with ADHD have other learning disabilities. Dyslexia, other learning disorders, and tic disorder are common conditions that can coexist with ADHD. Additional therapy may be necessary for these children with multiple diagnoses.

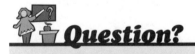 *Question?*

Can my child become addicted to ADHD medication?
Addiction is highly unlikely. The process of ADHD diagnosis and management is rigorous, and regular follow-up office visits ensure that any problem caused by the medication can be promptly detected and remedied.

The Rise of Autism

Autism has been a hotbed of debate on many fronts. Whether it is a discussion on vaccine safety or environmental pollutants, autism generates more emotional response than almost any other condition. Furthermore, as the incidence of autism is clearly rising, the most disconcerting thing is that no one knows what is causing the increase or why.

What Is Autism?

Children with autism find it difficult to interpret social and emotional cues from everyday social interactions. In addition, the majority of autistic children have various degree of communication deficit. Compared to their other intellectual skills, their language skills are usually significantly underdeveloped, which means that they may be smarter than they appear. Most autistic children score below average in IQ tests, but their true intellect is difficult to ascertain due to their linguistic limitations. In addition to problems with communication, many autistic children also have trouble adapting to changes in routine. Obsessive-compulsive tendencies are common in people with autism.

Diagnosing Autism

Most autistic children are diagnosed before the age of three, although many of them demonstrate some behavioral abnormalities at significantly younger ages. Most experts agree that the majority of autistic children have early signs of social and communicative difficulties before the age of one. You should consult your pediatrician about conducting additional evaluations of your child if you observe the following behavior:

- Lack of verbal communication (no vocabulary by the age of sixteen months)
- Infrequent eye contact
- Absence of hand gesture, such as pointing, by age one
- Lack of imaginative (or pretend) play

- Repeating certain jingles, such as those from television commercials or songs, in the wrong context
- Failure to respond to name when being directly addressed

There are standardized scoring charts that specifically aid the clinician in diagnosing autism. Your doctor may use one of these questionnaires to screen for autistic traits if your child is suspected of having autistic tendencies.

Asperger's Syndrome

Asperger's syndrome is a variant of autism. Children with Asperger's syndrome also face significant challenges in reading emotional cues or acting appropriately in social situations, but they have normal or near-normal language skills. Frequently, they come across as being rude or angry. Children with Asperger's syndrome frequently have specific obsessions within a narrow interest, and they object to deviation from routine.

What Causes Autism?

It is most frustrating that the medical community has not yet elucidated the cause of a condition as devastating as autism. What makes the matter even more urgent is that the incidence of autism appears to have increased within the past few decades. Genetics certainly plays an important role, but there are obviously other environmental and developmental factors that contribute to the onset of the condition. Siblings of autistic children are at a much higher risk of developing autism themselves. Relatives of autistic children are also more likely to have language problems or other minor communicative disorders.

As discussed in depth in Chapter 9, childhood immunizations are not the cause of autism. Several well-conducted studies have refuted any possible connection between vaccines and the triggering of autism or other related disorders. Though in the past it was believed that certain parenting styles could produce autistic tendencies in children, this hypothesis has also been disproved.

Treatment

Even though there is no cure for autism, behavioral and linguistic training have been extremely helpful in improving the functioning of autistic children. Many learn to interact appropriately in social situations and to live independently. Since autistic children frequently have other physical or psychiatric conditions that are associated with autism, including seizures, ADHD, and anxiety disorder, medications have a useful role in helping them adapt to the environment.

There are many unscrupulous individuals in the world who take advantage of parents' desperate search for a cure or treatment for autism. They often recommend expensive and unorthodox treatments with the promise of a dramatic improvement in behavior. It's truly unfortunate that there are so many who lack moral integrity and prey on the parents' desperation. Before you seek any alternative treatment, consult your child's doctor. You may save yourself a lot of money and false hope.

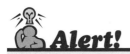

Alert!

Hyperbaric oxygen therapy and mega-doses of vitamin B have been touted as potential treatment for autism, but their validity has not been demonstrated by any scientific study. Before you put your child through any unproven therapy, talk to your doctor to confirm its efficacy and safety.

Children with Depression

Childhood depression is an underrecognized and underdiagnosed condition. Due to the stigma associated with mental illnesses in general, some parents are reluctant to seek help, even when they suspect that something may be wrong.

The earliest signs of depression in children include sudden changes in academic performance, changes in eating and sleeping habits, and significant fluctuation in weight. The child may appear to lose interest in the things that used to fascinate her. Excessive fatigue or irritability may also indicate the onset of depression.

If you suspect your child may be depressed and she is demonstrating the changes described above, you should seek the help of a mental-health professional immediately. There are many approaches to childhood depression. Some involve counseling and behavior treatment, while others involve the use of medication. A delay in treatment can have devastating consequences.

Anxiety Disorders in Children

Anxiety problems are often overlooked in children because many adults assume that the simple life of a child cannot possibly be stress inducing. However, many children do suffer from anxiety disorder, and they are vastly undertreated. A normal degree of anxiety is expected to occur from time to time when special circumstances arise in a child's life. For example, the birth of a sibling, the death of a pet, or the start of a new school all may induce elevated tension. It is important to distinguish a normal elevation in anxiety level from an excessive degree of anxiety that may be pathologic.

Typically, if the child's anxiety does not manifest itself in physical symptoms, it is usually within normal limits. In addition, anxiety should not prevent the child from participating in routine activities. If anxiety interrupts playtime or mealtime, it may be time for the parents to seek professional help. Several distinct anxiety disorders can be present in children, and the most common ones are described in this section.

Generalized Anxiety Disorder

Children with generalized anxiety disorder have such an elevated degree of anxiety that they find it impossible to control their worries. In addition, they may feel restless and irritable, which makes it difficult for them to focus. The anxiety may also interfere with sleeping and eating.

Separation Anxiety

Separation anxiety is a common childhood psychiatric condition. It is considered a normal part of childhood development when it occurs between the ages of six months and three or four years. Depending on the temperament of the individual child, anxiety may occur when the child is separated from the caregiver. Unless the intensity of the anxiety interferes with daily routine, it is not considered pathologic. School phobia is one form of separation anxiety, in which the child experiences an excessive degree of anxiety at school.

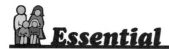

Essential

If your child is having a tough time enjoying playtime or adapting to the school environment, you may want to have him evaluated by a pediatric psychiatrist. Medication is usually not necessary, but it may be used in some cases.

Obsessive-Compulsive Disorder

Children are all unique, and personality differences certainly should not always be interpreted as abnormalities. However, children with obsessive-compulsive disorder have a hard time concentrating on their daily activities. Instead, their minds are preoccupied with intrusive thoughts and urges. They may act out these incessant thoughts by carrying out certain ritualistic acts. Most commonly, these involve a fear of dirt and germs. The fear of contamination causes them to wash their hands repeatedly, often to the point that they cannot get anything accomplished due to the amount of time they spend cleaning themselves.

Counseling may be effective for some children with obsessive-compulsive disorder, but there are also safe and effective medications that alleviate obsessive thoughts and acts. A mental-health professional is the best resource to consult for the management of this condition.

Post-Traumatic Stress Disorder

This is perhaps the most serious form of childhood anxiety disorder. Children who have witnessed abusive acts or have been victims themselves can become fearful of certain situations. Violent circumstances are certainly traumatic, and verbal or emotional abuse can be just as harmful to a child's pysche as physical abuse. Recurring thoughts of the event may intrude on the daily activities of these children, and avoidance of objects or situations that may remind them of the event is common.

If your child has gone through a serious traumatic event and is having a hard time getting over his fears, you should seek counseling right away. Medication may be helpful in reducing the anxiety level, but long-term counseling is usually also necessary for a permanent recovery.

CHAPTER 14

Attack of the Asthma

Affecting 5 million children in the United States, asthma is the most common chronic childhood illness. Asthmatic children are twice as likely to miss school as children without asthma. Asthma is also responsible for countless days of missed work because parents have to leave the job to care for their asthmatic children. Approximately half of children with asthma are restricted from some form of school activity due to their condition. It's a far-reaching problem that affects virtually everyone, and it imposes a tremendous burden on society.

Is It Asthma?

How do you know whether your child has asthma? Children often start showing signs of this problem while they are still very young, but asthma can strike at any age. Asthma can be difficult to diagnose. There is no simple blood test or X-ray that can be done to confirm a suspicion of asthma. A sophisticated lung-function test can diagnose the problem in adults, but it is impractical to administer to children. The vast majority of young asthmatic children are diagnosed exclusively by clinical manifestation. In other words, a collection of symptoms suggests that the condition is present.

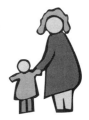

A Wheezy Proposition

Wheezing is a whistling sound that is produced by an asthmatic person who is breathing out. The wheezing sounds can be quite loud, or they may barely be audible without a doctor's stethoscope. Anyone can reproduce this wheezing sound by forcefully blowing air from the lungs with an open mouth. However, asthmatics frequently wheeze even when they are just breathing normally.

People generally associate wheezing with asthma, but that doesn't necessarily mean that any child who wheezes must have asthma. Many other conditions can cause wheezing, including a lung infection or an inhaled foreign object inside the lungs (such as a watermelon seed). Conversely, not everyone with asthma wheezes. Many children suffer from a form of asthma known as cough-variant asthma. These children rarely have wheezing when they have an asthma attack. Instead, they cough violently and repeatedly.

 Essential

If your child has a chronic cough, he may actually be having recurrent asthma attacks. As a good rule of thumb, if a cough lasts for more than two weeks, you should have your child checked out by a doctor. Other conditions, such as a sinus infection or nasal allergy, may also trigger a chronic cough.

Besides the coughing and wheezing it causes, asthma can also manifest itself as difficulty in breathing during exercise or as a sporadic nighttime cough. Some children may describe a sensation of tightness in their chests, or they might experience a coughing attack when they are laughing. Any of these symptoms may indicate the presence of asthma.

Asthma is strongly related to other allergic conditions. Skin allergy, commonly known as eczema, tends to run in the families of children with asthma and nasal allergy. As mentioned in Chapter 10, skin allergy, nasal allergy, and asthma make up the triad of allergic conditions that are strongly hereditary. Doctors call these three conditions the "atopic triad." Atopy is just a fancy medical word for allergy.

The heredity nature of atopy means that if one or both parents have these allergic conditions, the child has a greater chance of having asthma. If a sibling has allergy problems, the likelihood is also increased. This is why your pediatrician may inquire about the health history of other family members.

Trial of Medication

One of the best ways to confirm an asthma diagnosis based on clinical symptoms is to have your child try an asthma medication for a brief period of time (one to two weeks). If your child gets significant relief from an asthma medication, there is a strong probability that your child has asthma.

Even though it does not seem very scientific for a doctor to simply "try" a medication without first establishing a firm diagnosis, such a medication trial yields important information about the underlying reason for your child's symptoms. If the symptoms are completely unaffected by the asthma medication, then your child's chronic cough is most likely caused by something other than asthma.

Many parents are reluctant to let their child start using an asthma inhaler out of fear the child will never be able to stop. It is a common misconception that asthma medications are addictive. Another common belief is that once people start taking them, their lungs become dependent on the medications. Coming off the medications makes them suffer more because their lungs have been "weakened" by the asthma inhaler.

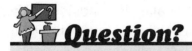

Question?

Can my child become addicted to his inhaler?
Many parents are afraid that once their child starts using an inhaler, he will become dependent on it. They fear that even if their child had no asthma problems before starting to use the inhaler, inhaler usage will ruin his lungs and transform him into an asthmatic. This worry is entirely unfounded.

Even though this belief is common, there is absolutely no basis for this way of thinking. Any physician will tell you that asthma inhalers are completely nonaddictive. These inhalers do not transform someone who is otherwise healthy into an asthmatic. As far as doctors are concerned, asthma is primarily a genetic condition. No one can develop asthma as a result of taking some medication. It's simply impossible. (See pages 206–210 for a complete discussion of asthma medications.)

Types of Asthma

To come up with a standard guideline for physicians to manage asthma, asthma experts nationwide have classified the breathing problem into various categories. This was necessary because the severity and manifestation of asthma often vary widely in different individuals. No single treatment plan is right for everyone. Doctors must tailor a patient's management plan and treatment goals based on the individual's needs and lifestyle.

Exercise-Induced Asthma
Children with exercise-induced asthma only have breathing trouble when they are engaged in strenuous activity. They do not have nighttime coughing or prolonged coughing spells when they catch a cold. This form of asthma is arguably the

mildest, but it still has the potential of causing severe breathing problems.

Since this pattern of asthma attack is more or less predictable, it can be most easily managed, if the parents and child understand when to use the medication and when to seek help from medical professionals. Most of these children do not need a daily maintenance dose of asthma medication, but exceptions are common based on individual needs.

Cough-Variant Asthma

Children suffering from cough-variant asthma do not necessarily wheeze when they have an asthma attack. Instead, they have a nagging cough that is often dry and forceful. Unlike a cough that can be triggered in anyone with a cold, a cough in a child with cough-variant asthma can last for more than a month. Besides being chronic, this asthma-related cough is often worse at night. During the day the child might not cough at all.

It is not always easy to distinguish cough-variant asthma from a cough triggered by a cold or bronchiolitis. Your child's pediatrician might try a brief course of asthma medication to make this distinction more clear.

Intermittent or Persistent

Asthma experts classify the severity of asthma according to how often symptoms manifest themselves. Children with mild asthma have symptoms no more than twice a month, but children with more severe asthma may experience cough or trouble breathing weekly or even daily.

Whether your child has chronic asthma or just mild occasional asthma needs to be determined by your child's pediatrician. There are many factors to be considered when making this decision, including how often your child coughs at night and whether your child suffers from breathing problems during increased activities. Your child's doctor will ask you these questions to determine whether long-acting medications need to be part of the asthma management regime. (These asthma medications are discussed at length on pages 206–210.)

What Causes Asthma?

One of the best ways to understand asthma is to compare it to nasal allergy. In reality, nasal allergy and asthma are the same condition occurring in two different places. Both nasal allergy and asthma are triggered by an overactive immune system, and both occur in parts of the body that are designed for breathing. The only difference is that the nose sits right on the face, so any irritation is plainly obvious. Asthma is basically an allergic reaction that occurs inside the lungs. It's more mysterious because the lungs are hidden deep inside the body. You can't see the result of the irritation easily.

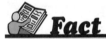 **Fact**

Children with asthma are more likely to suffer from nasal allergy and skin allergy. These conditions often occur in the same individual or in the same family. A good pediatrician will inquire about these other conditions when evaluating a child for asthma.

The symptoms of nasal allergy and asthma are directly comparable. With nasal allergy, the nose is often itchy and the sufferer sneezes frequently. For an asthmatic, coughing is basically sneezing of the lungs. For nasal allergy, congestion of the nose is a major manifestation. For asthma, chest tightness is the equivalent of congestion. For nasal allergy, the copious amount of discharge is often a major annoyance. For asthma, the "wet" cough that is full of phlegm is the corresponding nasal discharge.

As you can see, nasal allergy and asthma are closely related. In fact, an untreated nasal allergy is one of the most common triggers for asthma. This is the reason why it's so important to treat both nasal allergy and asthma when both conditions coexist in the same child. Otherwise, it is nearly impossible to adequately control asthma symptoms if the presence of nasal allergy is overlooked.

Drawing from the comparison above, which demonstrates that nasal allergy is irritation and inflammation of the nose, you should understand that asthma is an inflammatory condition as well. Inflammation is when a part of the body becomes raw and irritated. The result of inflammation is swelling, redness, and irritation of the tissue involved. Understanding inflammation is the key to understand asthma and its symptoms.

Asthma is inflammation inside the lungs, which means when an asthma attack occurs, it's not simply a problem with coughing and wheezing, but a problem with inflammation. Whenever the lung tissue becomes inflamed, it becomes swollen, irritated, and makes a lot of mucus.

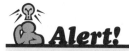

Alert!

You should not administer regular over-the-counter cough medications to your asthmatic child. These regular cough medications do not have any effect on the inflammation in the lungs. Temporarily suppressing the cough just delays the appropriate treatment for asthma.

It is important to view asthma as an inflammatory condition because this is fundamental to understanding the treatment strategy for asthma. It is inadequate to simply treat the cough. It is more important to suppress the inflammation inside the lungs. Without taking care of the inflammation, the short-term cough-suppressing medication just masks the danger beneath the surface.

Asthma Triggers

Parents must first learn the triggers for their child's asthma before they can effectively manage. The key to successful asthma management is to anticipate problems before they occur. Since each asthmatic is unique, parents have to learn the triggers the hard way—at least for the first episode for each trigger.

The Abominable Viruses

By far, cold viruses are the biggest culprits for triggering asthma attacks in children. Whenever your asthmatic child comes down with a cold, you must brace yourself and expect the worst from his asthma. It is usually a good idea to strike back preemptively by escalating the intensity of asthma medications at the earliest sign of a cold. Doing so could potentially prevent a disastrous asthma attack, one that could land your child in the emergency room or even in the hospital.

Exactly how you should increase the asthma medication needs to be directed by your child's pediatrician. Before asthma strikes, every asthmatic child needs to have a clear plan. Talk to your doctor if you don't have a very detailed counter-strike strategy to prevent severe asthma attacks.

 Essential

The best way to prevent colds is to encourage your child to develop the habit of frequent hand washing. It may seem old-fashioned, but this tried-and-true method is the most effective germ-prevention regimen known to modern science.

Prevention is far preferable to dealing with a crisis. If your child's asthma worsens with each cold, the best strategy is to avoid catching a cold in the first place.

Allergies as Triggers

The other common trigger for childhood asthma is nasal allergy. If your child has specific allergies that make his nose runny and congested, these allergens can trigger both the nasal allergy and asthma simultaneously.

The most common indoor allergens include dust and pet dander. These triggers can often be controlled to some degree, but there are exceptions. Parents can minimize the accumulation of dust inside the household but usually cannot eliminate it completely. Pets can be kept outdoors in the yard or at least outside of the child's bedroom. Making sure that nobody smokes is beneficial for everyone involved. Secondhand smoke is not only bad for asthma, it carries numerous other health risks as well.

Outdoor allergens are more difficult to avoid than indoor ones. Many children are allergic to pollens or grass. Since you cannot completely remove all vegetation from the neighborhood, the only effective way to avoid these outdoor allergens is to control the nasal allergy with medications.

Activity as Trigger

Most children with asthma experience shortness of breath when their activity level increases. While this is not universally true for pediatric asthmatics, it's common enough to cause a lot of problems for active children.

Many parents and teachers approach this type of asthma prevention the wrong way. They restrict the amount and type of activities these children can engage in because of their asthma condition. This is one of the worst things that can be done to these children.

These children need to participate in physical activities as much as anyone else does. They should never be held back because of their asthma. Instead of letting their asthma dictate what they can and cannot do, parents must use whatever medication they need so that these children can do anything their hearts desire. You should control your children's asthma so the asthma does not control their lives.

Coping with Asthma

If your child has chronic asthma symptoms, the most dangerous thing is not the chronic coughing but the chronic state of inflammation inside the lungs. When body tissues are chronically inflamed, they are gradually destroyed in the process. Chronic, uncontrolled asthma slowly destroys lung tissue. This is why chronic asthma must be controlled, not just for the sake of symptom relief but to save the lungs from permanent destruction.

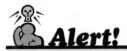

Alert!

The research studies that revealed that chronic inflammation of lung tissue slowly destroyed it came out more than ten years ago, and finally most of the doctors are becoming aware of this recommendation. If your doctor instructs your child to stay on an asthma control or maintenance medication, make sure to follow this direction to the letter.

Fortunately, this process of lung destruction by asthma occurs very slowly, and usually it does not happen unless the asthma is untreated for more than a decade. It's not too late to start your child on a control inhaler if she needs it.

Albuterol to the Rescue

There are two main types of medications used to treat asthma. One of them is known as the fast-acting "rescue" medicine. This medicine is called albuterol. It is dispensed in many forms, including a syrup, a liquid to be used with a machine, and an inhaler. Each form has its place in the management of asthma.

The syrup is easy to administer, especially to babies. It does not require additional medical equipment for its administration, and it's only given three times a day. However, this form of albuterol tends to be somewhat less effective, and its side effect of making the heart race is more pronounced. Doctors sometimes prescribe albuterol syrup when they treat a mild wheezing in infants. This is usually used for patients who do not have chronic asthma.

Another common way to administer albuterol is by using an inhaler. This method is by far the most popular. The albuterol is stored inside a small metallic aerosol canister, and the medicine sprays out when one end of the canister is depressed. It works similarly to a hair spray, except the canister is much smaller.

Any child using albuterol from an inhaler must use the inhaler in conjunction with a spacer. A spacer is nothing more than a plastic tube connected to a facemask (Aerochamber is a common commercial brand). The facemask covers the nose and mouth of the child. The inhaler is attached to the spacer from one end, and the mask is placed over the nose and mouth of the child from the other end. When albuterol sprays out from the canister, the air inside the spacer slows down the aerosolized albuterol particles. Without the spacer, the aerosolized particles travel at great speed, and most of the medication gets sprayed to the back of the mouth instead of traveling deep inside the lungs. Using an inhaler without attaching the spacer is quite useless.

 Essential

A common misconception is that albuterol administered via the nebulizer machine works better than the inhaler with a spacer. Even though this may appear to be true, this myth has been debunked by numerous well-conducted research studies. Nevertheless, doctors often face an uphill battle trying to convince parents otherwise.

Albuterol can also be given in the form of a liquid solution vaporized by a special machine. This machine is commonly referred to as a nebulizer. The albuterol solution is put inside the machine, and the machine nebulizes the albuterol into a mist. This mist is subsequently inhaled by the child.

The advantage of using a nebulizer is that it can be administered to very young infants or active toddlers who will not tolerate having the masked spacer on their faces. However, the medication cannot be given unless the machine is working. The machine is not very portable, and it needs an electrical outlet to function. These logistical limitations restrict its usefulness.

After an introduction to the various ways to administer albuterol, parents need to know when to use this medication. It is often called the "fast-onset" asthma medicine because it kicks in after about ten to fifteen minutes. Its effect lasts for two to four hours. During an asthma attack, it may need to be administered repeatedly to control the wheezing or coughing.

The way albuterol works is that it relaxes the lungs. Imagine someone suffering from nasal allergy as having an itchy nose. Well, children with asthma basically have "itchy" lungs. Albuterol temporarily takes this itchiness away and expands the lungs.

Steroid

Another major type of asthma medication is the steroid. This is a powerful drug that is more important for chronic asthmatics than albuterol. Steroids can be administered in three different ways as well, just like albuterol. The advantages and disadvantages of each method of administration are similar to those described for albuterol.

Inhaled steroids are used to control asthma on a long-term basis. They are frequently referred to as the "maintenance" asthma medication. Unlike albuterol, they do not work immediately after administration. In fact, it can take eight to twelve hours before they even start to work. For this reason, steroid inhalers cannot be used to relieve a sudden asthma attack. By the time they kick in, it may be too late to relieve your child with a severe asthma attack.

Even though inhaled steroids take a long time to kick in, they work wonders in extinguishing the inflammation caused by asthma when they are used over the long term. Because it is important to prevent lung inflammation at all times, these medications must be used daily in order to be effective. They are useless if used only sporadically or on an as-needed basis.

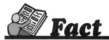

Fact

The steroid used to treat asthma and other inflammatory condition is not the same kind of steroid that some professional bodybuilders and athletes abuse. It is called corticosteroid. It does not make a person stronger but works instead to reduce inflammation. Using it will not give a girl masculine features.

It's a good analogy to compare the use of steroid inhalers to tooth brushing. You can't have your child brush her teeth only after she starts having a toothache. By the time she has a cavity, it's obviously too late to brush it away. Similarly, you can't wait until your child has an asthma attack to give her the inhaled steroid. By the time the asthma has flared up, the inflammation has already set in, and the damage done to the lung tissue has already occurred.

There are some new inhaled steroids that do not come in an aerosolized canister. One of the most popular ones is called Advair. This is actually a combination medication that includes both a steroid component and a long-acting form of albuterol. Advair is different from other inhalers in that the medication is sucked out of a plastic discus instead of being sprayed and inhaled. Unlike a traditional inhaler, this discus is not used with a spacer. However, not all children know how to suck the medication out of the dispenser. If your child can use the medication with the correct technique, this medication should be considered.

While it is crucial for chronic asthmatics to use inhaled steroids on a daily basis, doctors know that inhaled steroids can slow down vertical growth. However, this temporary reduction in height is small and transient. Since most children grow out of their asthma problem as they get older, it is likely that your child will stop using her steroid inhaler at some point in the future. Children who take inhaled steroids catch up on their height within six months to a year after the medication is stopped.

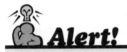

Alert!

There are many brands of steroid inhalers. The most common ones are Flovent and QVAR. These inhalers should be used to suppress the inflammation inside the lungs on a long-term basis. They do not work for a sudden asthma attack. For quick relief, use an albuterol inhaler instead.

Steroid syrup taken orally works similarly to the inhaled steroid, but it cannot be used on a long-term basis. Unlike inhaled steroids, oral steroid becomes absorbed into the body and travels everywhere. Even though this is by far the most potent form of steroid and it powerfully suppresses a severe asthma attack, it can also cause serious side effects if it is used for more than two weeks. It only has a short-term role in controlling severe asthma attack.

On very rare occasions, oral steroid is used to control severe chronic asthma on a long-term basis. All of these patients have asthma so severe that it does not respond to any other medication. Your child's doctor will weigh the benefits and risks of using oral steroid chronically. These children are the exceptions rather than the rule.

An Ounce of Prevention

The best way to avoid making frequent trips to the emergency room for treatment of asthma attacks is to anticipate problems before disaster strikes. It is the pediatrician's job to educate you and provide you with a detailed plan for managing your child's asthma. This plan needs to include ways to prevent asthma triggers, ways to suppress internal inflammation caused by asthma, and specific steps for what to do in case of a flare-up.

Having a Plan

Knowing what to expect and knowing what to do are crucial steps for parents in managing their child's asthma. Studies have shown that written instructions that detail a step-by-step plan in dealing with asthma attacks are the most effective way to stop sudden asthma exacerbations. Most asthma specialists endorse using such a written asthma-treatment plan.

No one child reacts to his asthma the same way. Therefore, it is critical for each asthmatic to have a unique plan that is tailored to his own needs. If your doctor does not provide such written instructions, politely request them. Not only can preparation like this prevent you from making frequent trips to the emergency room, it can sometimes mean the difference between life and death.

Frequently, it is insufficient for just the parents to be familiar with the medications. It is not uncommon for grandparents or babysitters to be primarily responsible for taking care of the child during the day. They must be thoroughly instructed in the asthma plan as well. Finally, if the child is mature enough to learn about her own asthma regimen, she must start taking on the responsibility of knowing what to do. No one is better positioned to monitor and treat asthma problems than the asthma sufferer herself.

Avoiding Triggers

Knowing your child's asthma triggers and avoiding them are the first steps toward a successful asthma-management program. If frequent asthma attacks can be prevented, parents won't have to resort to activating the emergency plan very often. Keeping your child away from environmental triggers is important. If avoidance is not feasible, you can at least beef up the maintenance medication to hopefully ward off a potential asthma exacerbation.

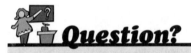

Question?

Will my child ever outgrow her asthma?
The answer to this question is more complicated than a simple yes or no. Most children with asthma flare-ups that are triggered by a cold or exercise tend to improve as they reach adolescence. However, given that many adults have asthma, this obviously does not happen to everyone.

If your child suffers from activity-induced attacks, make sure that he carries his quick-acting inhaler with him when he's participating in sports. Ten to fifteen minutes prior to engaging in activities, he should administer two puffs of albuterol from the inhaler. Not only can this measure prevent an asthma attack, it can also allow your child to attain his maximal athletic performance without being hindered by asthma.

CHAPTER 15
All about Allergies

I f you think that there are more children suffering from allergies today than in the past, you are correct. Even though scientists do not have a perfect explanation for the increase in allergies, allergic conditions affect more children than ever before. With this significant rise in childhood allergies, parents are increasingly frustrated with this problem. Luckily, parents and doctors are armed with better and safer medications to control allergies.

What Are Allergies?

The public and mass media use the term "allergy" loosely. Without a clear definition, a lot of confusion and miscommunication can result. From a medical and scientific perspective, allergy is a condition in which the immune system reacts to something in the environment that is harmless.

The human immune system is an incredible thing. Its job is primarily to protect the human body from infections. You can imagine the immune system as the defense department of the body. When the body is under siege by microbes, the immune system sends out microscopic troops to ward off an invasion. Without an intact immune system, human beings would be constantly threatened by various infections.

However, having a large army of elite troops can be a double-edged sword. Sometimes the armed forces sound a false alarm and respond to an innocuous material from the environment. This response could be a localized mobilization, or it could be a full-scale assault on a nonexistent enemy. When the immune system reacts inappropriately to a benign target, the body experiences an allergic reaction.

While the topic of allergy is broad and encompasses skin allergies, asthma, hay fever, and other less common conditions, the discussion in this chapter is limited to nasal allergies and reaction to food or chemicals. It is worth mentioning here that skin allergy (commonly known as eczema), nasal allergy, and asthma are closely related conditions. These three conditions are all caused by an overactive immune system, and they tend to run within the same family. If Uncle Bob has nasal allergy and Grandpa has asthma, your child may be cursed with eczema. They are all really different manifestations of the same hypersensitive immune system.

Popular Misconceptions of Allergy

The nonmedical community often uses the word "allergy" to mean a variety of reactions to environmental exposures. For example, a lot of people believe that they are "allergic" to milk because they experience bloating, stomachache, and diarrhea after consuming dairy products. Others claim that their child is "allergic" to juice because she develops diarrhea after consuming a large quantity of it. Neither of these situations describes a true allergic condition because neither reaction involves the immune system.

In the first scenario, the reaction to dairy products described is most commonly due to lactose intolerance. These individuals lack the ability to digest the sugar in milk, so every time they consume any dairy product, the large amount of undigested sugar inside their intestine triggers a bunch of unpleasant feelings. This reaction involves the digestive system, not the immune system. In the second case, drinking excessive fruit juices over-whelms the intestine with sugar. Once again, this undigested sugar wreaks havoc in the body.

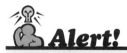

Alert!

True lactose intolerance in babies is exceedingly rare. Most lactose-intolerant children and adults develop their intolerance in later child-hood. Babies are almost universally capable of digesting sugar in milk. Ask your pediatrician so you don't switch unnecessarily to one of the expensive specialized formulas.

Unfortunately, the industry is quick to take advantage of these common misconceptions. They make lactose-free for-mula for babies who are allegedly "allergic" to milk, when in fact most of these babies have run-of-the-mill baby reflux. The lactose-free formula makes absolutely no difference in these babies' symptoms. Of course, these specialized formulas cost more than the regular kind, and anxious parents who purchase these special formulas spend more than they need to in the false belief they are doing more to keep their child healthy.

Allergy to Cigarette Smoke

Many people avoid cigarette smoke because they think they are allergic to it. Even though this is not really true, it isn't a bad idea after all. Secondhand smoke is extremely dangerous and toxic. Even though smoke from cigars and cigarettes cannot trigger an allergic reaction in people, everyone should avoid it like the plague. When people experience a burning sensation in their nose and eyes in the vicinity of smokers, they are being irritated by the microscopic smoke particles. This reaction does not involve the immune system, so it is not considered an aller-gic reaction.

More Allergic than Ever

More children suffer from allergy in today's world than ever before. Their constant suffering from runny noses and teary eyes begs the question—what is the reason behind the increased prevalence of allergic conditions? Many theories attempt to answer this question, but the most popular and accepted explanation is based on the observation that people tend to live in a cleaner environment than in the past.

What is meant by "clean" is not that today's environment is less polluted or that the air people breathe is fresher. On the contrary, humanity is worse off in those aspects than in the past. However, most people do live in an environment in which they have less interaction with wild animals and livestock. Most people also have less direct contact with human and animal feces.

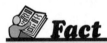 *Fact*

A famous study published in the *Journal of the American Medical Association* in 2002 found that children growing up with at least two pets in the household tend to have fewer allergic problems later in life than children without any pets. It is theorized that having more pets around exposes these children to the bacteria in the feces of the animals, which makes these children less prone to allergic conditions.

This hypothesis is based on the idea that the immune system can do one of two things. It can either protect the body from infections, or it can trigger allergic reactions. If the immune system is preoccupied with fighting off infections, it does not have the spare resources to cause allergies. For children with multiple pets, the additional burden on the immune system to ward off a higher level of bacteria prevented their immune system from triggering allergic reactions. It's kind of like teenage boys.

If they don't have a structured after-school program to occupy their time, they'll be up to no good.

Be aware, though, that this theory is far from being proven. It's an interesting concept, and it's certainly plausible, but applying this way of thinking to the real world is jumping the gun. The message from this study is that having multiple pets in a household with young children might not be such a bad thing. Ultimately, scientists may use this knowledge and come up with new ways of treating or preventing allergies.

Food Allergies

There are probably more myths surrounding food allergies than any other types of allergic reaction. Food is essential for survival, and for a sufferer of food allergy, every meal may represent a trip to the emergency room or an embarrassing way to end a first date.

But food allergies are no laughing matter. A reaction could range from a minor rash to a full-blown anaphylactic reaction, where the entire body swells up. Allergy has the potential to be a silent and quick killer.

The Notorious Gang of Eight

To some degree, it has become almost "cool" to have a food allergy. While food allergy can be a serious medical condition, being allergic to food has infiltrated the pop culture. Sometimes it seems that everyone has a trendy food allergy.

Food allergy actually isn't as common as you may think. A national survey indicates that close to 30 percent of Americans believe that they have an allergy to food. However, most medical studies estimate that no more than 5 percent of the general population has an actual food allergy. This falsely elevated reporting results from the confusion of many nonallergic reactions with true food allergies.

It is quite surprising that a small number of food items cause the majority of food allergies. The most common culprits are these:

- Peanuts
- Tree nuts (walnuts, pecans)
- Eggs
- Milk
- Soy
- Wheat
- Fish
- Shellfish

While virtually any food can trigger allergy, these eight are responsible for most of the reactions.

Simply having a bad reaction to something she ate doesn't necessarily mean that your child has an allergy to some kind of food. It could be a case of food poisoning, where the actual food item is not to blame. The actual culprit for the allergic reaction could be difficult to tease out, since children rarely ingest a single food item at a time. If you suspect an allergic reaction, talk to your child's pediatrician to confirm or refute the suspicion. Additional blood tests may be necessary to medically diagnose a food allergy.

 Essential

A common myth regarding food allergy involves the notorious monosodium glutamate (MSG). This is a common additive to foods served in many Chinese restaurants. Its purpose is to enhance the flavor of the food. Even though there are numerous anecdotal reports of bad reactions to this compound, scientific studies have discredited the existence of a true allergic reaction to MSG.

Some individuals are extremely sensitive to food allergens. Even a trace amount of the food can trigger a life-threatening reaction. Occasional case reports have revealed that even cookware used to prepare peanut products can cross-contaminate another dish, even though the dish does not contain any peanut. Steam from shellfish inhaled by susceptible individuals has triggered anaphylactic reaction. If your child has severe reactions to food, you must be constantly vigilant to avoid exposure to the allergen.

It is possible for children to outgrow their food allergies, but this is mostly true for only egg and milk allergy. Most children with peanut allergy are going to be allergic to it for the rest of their lives. Since reaction to peanuts tends to be severe, it is wise to stay away from peanuts forever once a serious reaction occurs.

The best way to avoid developing food allergy is by postponing the introduction of solid foods to your baby until after six months of age. Numerous studies have proven the link between early introduction of solid foods and the development of food allergies later in life. Beside this additional risk, most babies younger than four months cannot hold their heads up to be fed with a spoon anyway.

Contrary to popular beliefs, maternal diet during pregnancy plays no role in the development of food allergy in babies. A large, well-conducted Swedish study published in the *Journal of Allergy and Clinical Immunology* in 1992 confirms the lack of association between maternal diet during pregnancy and the onset of childhood allergy for the unborn child.

When introducing a food to your baby for the first time, it is a good idea not to try another new food in the next four days. This way, if your baby has an allergic reaction to the food item, it is easy to figure out which food is the culprit. For older children, parents should delay introduction of peanut products, fish, and shellfish until after the age of three.

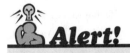
Alert!

If your child has a medically diagnosed severe food allergy, always carry emergency medication. This medication is basically injectable adrenaline. It is a potent antidote to a severe allergic reaction that involves the whole body. Having this medication nearby in case of a severe allergic reaction could mean the difference between life and death.

Even though food allergies in other family members do increase the likelihood of allergy in an individual, the direct inheritance of food allergies is not common. Even if both parents are severely allergic to peanuts, their child is most likely not going to share that same allergy. Pediatricians do not automatically test such a child for peanut allergy or assume that the child is allergic to peanuts. It is still a good idea, however, to closely monitor the child the first time he tries a peanut butter sandwich.

Pet Allergies

Many pet lovers would rather suffer from allergies (or have their spouse suffer) than to get rid of their pets. Not only do pets provide companionship, they are as important to some families as children. They are truly the pride and joy of their owners.

Unfortunately, many owners and their family members suffer allergic reactions to these beloved members of the family. These reactions range from mild nasal congestion, watery eyes, and repetitive sneezing to severe breathing difficulties. Sensitive individuals can stop breathing within minutes after an exposure to cat dander.

Sources of Pet Allergy

Children can be allergic to pets for many reasons. The most common sources of allergy include the skin of the animal, their saliva, and their urine. Contrary to common beliefs, pet hair is not a significant source of allergy for most people. The feathers and scales of some pets are also sources of allergy.

Pet dander, the skin that flakes off from animals, is one of the most potent sources of allergy. Dander is microscopic and can travel anywhere in a house through air currents. Even after a pet is removed from the house, the dander can remain in the house for up to seven months. This is the reason why a new homeowner or a new apartment tenant may experience severe allergy to a pet of the previous dweller.

Avoidance Measures

Even though the best advice to treat a pet allergy is to get rid of the pets, this is not always an acceptable option for many pet owners. Some allergists recommend switching to fish instead of cats or dogs. This substitution is a mere joke for most cat and dog lovers. There simply is no replacement for their beloved furry friends.

If you must have pets around the house, there are still things you can do to minimize allergic reaction in your children. Simply having the pets stay in the yard is a huge improvement. If this is unacceptable for you, perhaps you can at least keep the pets out of the child's bedroom or limit the animal to a single room inside the house. It's not a perfect solution, but it's better than having the pet spending the night in bed with the child.

 Essential

Many people believe that having shorthaired pets reduces their chance of developing allergies. This is largely a myth. However, hairy animals may trigger more allergic reactions if they are not washed frequently. Longer hairs tend to trap more dust and bacteria, which could cause allergic reactions on their own.

Obviously, if your child has a severe and life-threatening allergic reaction to your pet, such as breathing difficulties, giving the pet up for adoption is absolutely necessary. But remember, the pet dander may stay inside the house for up to seven months after the animal leaves, so don't expect an immediate resolution of allergic symptoms once the pet is gone.

Allergy Testing

Every parent of an allergic child is anxious to find out all the things in the world that the child is allergic to. That's why allergy testing is one of the most common requests parents make of their pediatricians. Before jumping the gun and ordering a bunch of tests, parents must understand how these tests are used and interpreted. Misinterpreting the results can actually do more harm than good.

The Skin Scratch Test

To figure out the potential for various food allergies, the skin prick test is one of the most common methods of determining sources of allergy. One of the advantages of performing skin tests is that the result is immediately available. The test can be quickly performed in the doctor's office, and it is not necessary to get any blood drawn at a lab.

To conduct this test, the doctor scratches the skin lightly with a needle and then places a small amount of purified allergen extract onto the scratched skin surface. If the child has an allergy to the item under scrutiny, the skin swells up and becomes red and itchy.

Your doctor should explain to you that prior to undergoing skin allergy testing, your child must refrain from using any oral antihistamines for at least one day. The test must be performed under the supervision of a physician who can handle an emergency in case a severe allergic reaction results from the scratch test. Most importantly, the skin test results must be interpreted by an experienced allergy expert. Misinterpreting the results can have a detrimental effect on your child. Most pediatricians prefer consulting an allergy specialist for such an evaluation.

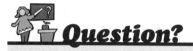 ***Question?***

When should my child be tested for food allergies?
Skin testing may be warranted if a severe allergic reaction has occurred and your doctor strongly suspects that food is the culprit. Indiscriminant testing without considering an individual's clinical history can only result in misdiagnosis and unnecessary dietary restrictions.

The Blood Test

While skin allergy testing is considered superior and more reliable than allergy testing through the blood, the advantage of a blood test is that the result is generally easier to interpret. Any experienced pediatrician can order and interpret the result of allergy blood tests without consulting an allergy specialist. Another advantage of performing the blood test is that patients do not have to stop taking antihistamines before the test is performed. Oral antihistamines (or any other medications, for that matter) do not influence the result of allergy blood tests. Finally, there is no risk for the child of a severe anaphylactic reaction when this test is performed.

There are some inherent limitations of blood allergy testing. People may test positive for certain types of food when they in fact do not have allergy to those food items. This false-positive result would lead them to avoid these foods unnecessarily. The results of blood allergy testing also take a lot longer to come back, compared to the immediacy of skin testing.

Misinterpretation of Results

No matter what type of allergy testing is desired, it is essential that the test results be interpreted correctly. Most general pediatricians and family practice physicians do not have the expertise or clinical experience to properly interpret the results of skin allergy tests. Misinterpreted results may remove many foods unnecessarily from your child's menu. More seriously, incorrect interpretation could lead to a false sense of security and expose your child to potential dangerous sources of food allergy.

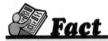 **Fact**

There is a common misconception that toddlers and infants are too young to be candidates for allergy testing. Even though infants younger than twelve months might have a less intense skin reaction to the allergen challenge, a skin allergy test can still be reliably performed and interpreted. It is usually performed under the supervision of an allergy specialist.

On the other hand, many general physicians are supremely qualified to evaluate the results of blood tests for food allergy. Politely ask your doctor about his experience with other children with food allergy. Your doctor will probably refer your child to an allergy expert if he does not feel comfortable interpreting these results himself.

Allergy Treatments

Children with chronic nasal allergy frequently do not seek relief from the symptoms. Even though these symptoms can be severe and debilitating, these children often suffer from the allergy chronically. They get used to the discomfort and accept the misery as part of their existence, and they might not even realize the possibility of a life free of allergy.

This does not mean that their quality of life does not suffer as a result of their allergy. More often than not, they do not get a restful sleep at night due to nasal congestion. As a result, they are chronically tired and feel drowsy during the day. Their mood might suffer, not to mention the potential effect on their academic performance. The role of the parents is to recognize these symptoms and bring them to the attention of the pediatrician. An astute pediatrician will notice some physical findings during the examination, but it is always better to alert the doctor to this concern.

Why Seek Treatment?

Allergy sufferers experience a lower quality of life, but this is not the only negative impact on their lives. Children with untreated nasal allergy also suffer from more ear and sinus infections. Recurrent ear infections can cause hearing loss and speech delay, both of which can hamper a successful life.

Lack of a good night's sleep can also make a child more prone to accidents. This could translate into serious bodily harm or injury to others. Chronic suffering from nasal congestion and sleep deprivation also influences emotion and mood.

Nasal Sprays

Numerous clinical studies have proven that prescription steroid nasal sprays are by far the most effective medications for curbing nasal allergy. Not only do they work well, they also have fewer side effects because the medication remains largely inside the nose. Unlike antihistamines such as Benadryl or Claritin, these medications are not used orally, so they are not absorbed into the bloodstream and delivered all over the body.

To derive the maximum benefit from the nasal spray, your child must use it on a daily basis. Again, you could compare using the spray to brushing your teeth. You know you shouldn't brush your teeth only after you start having a toothache. By the time the pain starts, you have probably already gotten a cavity and it's too late to brush the cavity away. Similarly, you shouldn't wait until your child has a severe allergic attack to use the nasal spray. In fact, it takes the nasal spray an average of four to six days before it takes effect. It is not a medication that can be used as needed. Parents must constantly remind their allergic child and ensure that he stays on the medication during the allergy season.

Some parents are concerned about using these steroid sprays because they fear the effect of steroids on their children. This worry is unfounded because the steroid in these sprays stays in the nose only. Only an extremely minute quantity is absorbed into the body. At such low levels, the steroid cannot affect your child's hormone level in any way.

The only side effect from these nasal sprays is the possibility of an occasional nosebleed. The trick to avoiding this problem is to aim the snout of the spray container away from the middle part of the nose. Do not insert the snout of the container too far into the nostrils. If your child still experiences nosebleeds, you can try using the nose spray every other day instead of daily. This side effect can be successfully prevented in almost every child.

Antihistamines

Despite the promises of the pharmaceutical companies, new-generation antihistamines such as Claritin (generic lorata-dine) are not very effective at alleviating the symptoms of nasal allergy. It is true that they do not cause drowsiness, unlike the older generation antihistamines (such as Benadryl), but they also don't do much in reducing allergic symptoms. Compared with steroid nasal sprays, they are far less effective in relieving nasal congestions and sneezing.

However, these medications do have a role in managing allergic conditions. Unlike the nasal sprays, they are either dis-pensed in liquid form or as a tablet that melts in the mouth. Some children may not allow you to spray anything up their nose, but they might be more willing to drink a liquid medication. Secondly, because these are taken orally, they are absorbed into the body and have an effect all over. If your child experiences itchy and watery eyes in addition to nasal symptoms, your doctor might consider using oral antihistamines instead of nasal sprays to control all the symptoms together. It is also acceptable in many situations to use the antihistamine medications in conjunction with nasal sprays.

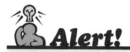

Alert!

Even though oral antihistamines tend to have a sedating effect on most children, some children can experience the exact opposite effect. Instead of feeling sleepy, they may become agitated and cranky after taking these medicines. Keep this possibility in mind before you administer these medications for their sleep-inducing properties.

Allergy Shots

Allergy shots are also called immunotherapy in the medical field. This process works by gradually exposing the immune system to small amounts of allergic material so that the body eventually gets used to the offending allergen. This sounds good on paper, but it doesn't always work that well in real life.

First and foremost, parents who are considering taking their children for allergy shots must understand the time and financial commitment required in this treatment regimen. To even contemplate a successful treatment, the total length of time for immunotherapy is between three and five years. Parents must take their child for frequent shots, ranging from twice a week to twice a month, and must keep this schedule religiously or the therapy will not work.

Secondly, the parents must have realistic expectations. On average, only a third of children who undergo allergy shots are free from their allergy, while the allergic problem for the rest of the children may stay the same or even get worse. Certainly, immunotherapy isn't the magic bullet for allergy, despite its tremendous time and resource commitment.

That said, allergy shots could be your child's best chance of remaining allergy free for an extended period of time or even for life. This promise of hope is certainly the attraction for thousands of parents who are willing to put themselves and their children through this grueling process.

CHAPTER 16

Vitamins and Supplements

Vitamins are often perceived as the cure-all for any medical condition. Not only are they touted for their ability to prevent illnesses, but other miraculous properties are also purported by their manufacturers. Unfortunately, many parents fall victim to these schemes and believe that their children will be seriously harmed if deprived of these alleged essential supplements. It is time for a medical professional to set the record straight.

Vital Amines

Vitamins were first found to be essential for human health by Dr. William Fletcher in 1905. The term "vitamin" was subsequently coined by the Polish scientist, Cashmir Funk, by combining the word "vital" and "amine."

Certain types of vitamin deficiency used to be common, and the scientific and medical communities were highly interested in these compounds. Over the years, the medical community has gained valuable knowledge about the roles vitamins play in the body's normal functions. Your child only needs a very small trace of vitamins to satisfy the body's daily requirement. Any excessive vitamins are simply excreted from the body.

Scientists have grouped vitamins into two categories: water-soluble and fat-soluble. These group-

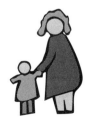

ings are not arbitrary. Instead, they have important implications on how the body absorbs and eliminates these chemicals.

Water-Soluble Vitamins

The water-soluble vitamins include vitamins in the B complex and vitamin C. Vitamin B consist of a collection of compounds, including thiamin (B1), riboflavin (B2), pyridoxine (B6), folic acid, and cobalamin (B12). These substances readily dissolve in water, so the body doesn't have the ability to store them. They are constantly being flushed out. As a result, your child must regularly consume small amounts of the water-soluble vitamins to prevent deficiency.

 Essential

One of the most important discoveries that has come out of vitamin research is that folic acid deficiency during pregnancy can significantly increase the risk of certain types of birth defects. These birth defects common involve deformity of the spinal cord or the brain.

The famous scientist Linus Pauling made vitamin C infamous by associating high doses of it with prevention of the common cold. Vitamin C deficiency, scurvy, is often associated with sailors because prolonged sea voyages often include no fresh fruits or vegetables in the diet. However, unless your child doesn't eat any vegetables or fruits at all, this vitamin deficiency is quite rare.

Fat-Soluble Vitamins

Fat-soluble vitamins include vitamins A, D, E, and K. These vitamins can be stored in fat tissues, so the body is less likely to run out of these vitamins even if your child doesn't consume them on a daily basis.

Vitamin A is crucial for maintenance of good skin and generation of the light-sensitive components of the eyes. Deficiency can lead to skin rashes and poor vision. Fresh fruits and vegetables are the best sources of vitamin A. Overdose of vitamin A is the most common vitamin overdose, and the result can be devastating. Excessive intake of vitamin A can cause severe headache and even death.

Vitamin D is essential in the absorption of calcium and building strong bones. Rickets is a form of vitamin D deficiency in which the bones become extremely soft due to the lack of calcium. Vitamin D deficiency is still common in today's world. Natural sunlight plays an important role in enabling the body to produce its own vitamin D.

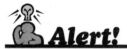

Alert!

Dark-skinned children and adults are especially susceptible to vitamin D deficiency because the high concentration of skin pigmentation blocks sunlight from penetrating the body. People living in higher latitudes are also at higher risk of becoming vitamin D deficient because of the relative reduction in sun exposure.

Vitamin E is found in fresh vegetables and nuts. Early studies had demonstrated vitamin E's protective effect in preventing heart diseases and cancer, but more recent research has revealed that this connection is tenuous. Deficiency in vitamin E is extremely rare.

Vitamin K is an important factor in clotting. Without adequate vitamin K, the body's ability to stop bleeding is impaired. All newborns are naturally low in vitamin K, which is the rationale behind universal injection of vitamin K right at birth.

Redundant Supplementation

While vitamins are important for proper operation of the human body, a well-balanced diet rich in vegetables and fruits provides more than enough of the daily requirement of vitamins. Taking additional vitamins is mostly a superfluous endeavor that wastes time and money. In certain circumstances, taking excessive amount of vitamins may even be harmful to your child's health.

Who Needs Vitamin Supplements?

Only a select group of people need to take vitamin supplements. This small population includes pregnant women, breastfeeding mothers, premature infants, older individuals, and children with specific medical conditions, such as cystic fibrosis and other rare digestive disorders. Some people need special vitamin supplementation while they're taking certain types of medications, such as isoniazid (a medication used to treat tuberculosis). Your physician will recommend and prescribe such vitamins when the situation warrants it.

The official statement from the American Dietetic Association should send a clear message to all parents: "The best nutritional strategy for promoting optimal health and reducing the risk of chronic disease is to wisely choose a wide variety of foods." Dieticians do not recommend supplemental vitamins, and neither do doctors.

While medical professionals do not recommend that children follow a strict vegetarian diet, some cultural and religious practices make this type of diet necessary. It is possible to maintain a balanced intake of nutrients while following these restrictive diets, but it takes a wealth of nutritional knowledge and advanced menu planning to achieve it. If your child is a strict vegetarian, consult your doctor or a dietician before starting vitamin supplementation.

Too Much of a Good Thing

Just because vitamins are essential for the body doesn't mean your child should take a lot of them. Too much of a good thing can be a bad thing. Most pediatricians do not recommend that healthy growing children take a daily dose of vitamins. Just as excessive water can damage your brain, excessive amounts of vitamins can cause serious toxicity.

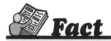 **Fact**

Scientist Linus Pauling promoted the belief that 75 percent of all cancers could be cured or prevented by high doses of vitamin C. No scientific studies have ever confirmed this hypothesis. He also claimed that by taking large quantities of vitamin C, people could cut their chance of catching a common cold in half. This belief has never been endorsed by any reputable scientific or medical organization.

For instance, taking too high a dose of vitamin A can cause swelling of the brain and death. Excessive amounts of vitamin C can trigger the formation of kidney stones. You should never indiscriminately supplement your child's diet with vitamins, especially when you are using more than one vitamin source.

Lack of Regulation

You might expect the government to have a tight control over vitamins and other supplementations sold in health-food stores, but this is not the case. Vitamins are technically not medications, so the FDA does not have jurisdiction over their safety and distribution. What makes the matter even worse is that these supplements can be obtained without a prescription, so misuse (either unintentional or purposeful) can run rampant.

Most of these supplements do not undergo the vigorous clinical testing that all prescription medications are required to go through before they receive government approval. Furthermore, their purity and efficacy are not regulated at all. Some may be overly potent, while others can lack any active ingredient.

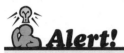

Alert!

Just because these supplements are not medications does not mean they are harmless. Many supplements are proven to be able to alter chemicals in the brain and elevate blood pressure. Some herbal supplements can be just as potent as prescription medications, and their effects may be harmful for some children.

Due to this lack of oversight, most pediatricians do not recommend that children take over-the-counter vitamins. If your child has a medical condition that requires him to take additional vitamins, the physician will actively prescribe them to you. It's not worth the risk to take chances with these unregulated chemicals.

Appetite Stimulants

Taking vitamins as an appetite stimulant is an extremely popular practice among parents. A corollary to this belief is that vitamins can stimulate growth and improve strength. All of these beliefs are pure nonsense.

Some believe that the more vitamins they give to their children, the more these children will grow. But providing vitamins to your children is just like watering a plant. More water doesn't necessarily mean better growth. In fact, overwatering a plant will eventually kill it. If a plant is already getting enough water, an excess of water will do no good. If your child is already getting all her vitamins and nutrients from a balanced diet, additional vitamins are just redundant and potentially even harmful.

 Essential

Many parents rationalize that because their children are picky eaters, they must supplement food with vitamins to make up for the poor intake of fruits and vegetables. This type of thinking is not only wrong but also dangerous. Taking vitamin supplements does not replace the need to eat fresh fruits and vegetables. Vitamins in pill form are an inadequate substitute for the real thing.

Vitamins do not help your child gain weight. Only additional caloric intake can increase body mass. Vitamins simply help the body function properly. You can compare them to credit cards. Like credit cards, vitamins make chemical transactions in the body easier and faster. Without them, the body cannot conduct business in many situations. However, the credit cards themselves do not make you richer. They just assist the transaction along the way.

If your child is underweight, she needs to consume more foods and calories. Throwing vitamins or other supplements at her won't do her any good.

Iron Will

Popeye the Sailor perpetuates the notion that iron supplementation is not only desired but necessary to enrich one's body. The cartoon character was originally conceived to encourage children's intake of green leafy vegetables, but this message got distorted in the cartoon caricature. Chronic iron deficiency can cause fatigue, but an excess of it does not provide anyone with super-human strength.

The Other Red Meat

While spinach does contain iron, the best source of dietary iron is meat. The form of iron in meat is more readily available for children to absorb. While red meats do contain a high level of iron, other lean meats, such as chicken or pork, are also great sources of iron.

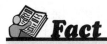 *Fact*

Contrary to common belief, seafood is a great source of iron. Oysters, salmon, and tuna are some of the best iron-rich foods. Many nuts also contain high levels of iron. You do not have to force your child to finish that bloody steak in order to make sure he gets enough iron in his diet after all.

For some strange reason, chicken is frequently considered not to be a type of animal meat. Parents often lament to doctors that their children do not eat any meat and that they only eat chicken. This fundamental paradox is hard to explain, but it's extremely common. Chicken is definitely a good source of iron, with the added benefit of containing less fat than beef or pork. Perhaps Popeye should have been chugging canned chicken or tuna instead of spinach.

Iron and Constipation

It is indeed true that an iron supplement can cause constipation, but iron-rich foods or iron-fortified foods seldom have this unpleasant side effect. Nevertheless, the myth linking iron and hard stools is solidly stuck in the public mind.

Iron-fortified infant formulas do not cause constipation. This is an extremely common myth that is widely believed by many parents and even medical professionals. Many parents falsely blame iron-containing formula for their baby's constipation, which makes them switch to a low-iron variety. Low-iron baby formula is extremely dangerous to an infant's health.

If your baby needs to take iron supplements because she is anemic, you can lower the probability of your baby experiencing constipation by dividing the daily dose and giving these smaller portions two or three times a day. Administering the iron supplement with food and increasing the intake of high-fiber foods and water may also reduce constipation. Do not stop the iron supplement if your child requires it.

Addressing Anemia

Anemia is a condition that often strikes without any outward manifestations, which could be why so many parents lose sleep over it. It's perceived as the hidden malady, slowly but constantly shaving away your child's intellect and physical potential.

The truth is that anemia is not as ominous as most parents fear. While chronic severe anemia can and does affect some children, most anemic children have a borderline blood count that does not pose a serious threat to their health.

Background and Definition

The red blood cells are responsible for carrying oxygen around the body. When your child's red blood cell concentration falls below a critical threshold, your child becomes anemic. The normal range for the concentration of red blood cells in the body varies according to the age of the child.

Newborn babies have a very high concentration of red blood cells because they needed to extract oxygen from the mother's blood before they were born. Once babies start to acquire oxygen using their own lungs, the additional blood cells are rendered redundant. The blood count quickly drops during the first month, but this is a normal phenomenon.

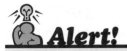

Alert!

Commercial infant formulas that contain low iron do not provide enough iron for growing infants. These formulas are extremely dangerous and should always be avoided. Prolonged use of these low-iron formulas can lead to severe and life-threatening anemia in babies.

Over the next few months after birth, the baby's primary source of iron is either breast milk or commercial formulas. While these sources of iron are not completely sufficient to sustain growth indefinitely, they are adequate for the first six months of life. After six months, it is important for your baby to start taking some solid foods and obtaining additional sources of iron from her diet.

The blood-cell concentration reaches its lowest point at around six months of age. As the child grows, the blood count gradually rises until it reaches the peak level of an adult. During puberty, testosterone boosts the blood level of boys. As a consequence, the typical blood-cell concentration for a mature man is higher than a woman's. This gender discrepancy is not seen prior to adolescence.

During pregnancy, all women become relatively anemic. Not only does the baby steal iron from the mother's body, the increased water retention and blood volume during pregnancy dilute the existing blood cells so the concentration falls. This is the rationale behind iron supplementation during pregnancy. Fortunately, this mild degree of anemia does not usually cause any harm to the mother or the baby.

Manifestation of Anemia

Most children with mild anemia do not have any external visible findings. Many parents believe that white spots on the face or dry skin indicates the presence of anemia, but neither of these physical findings is related to anemia. The most common cause of these pale spots on the face is eczema, which is an allergic skin condition described in Chapter 10.

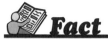**Fact**

Pale skin is usually a result of genetics and a lack of skin pigmentation rather than anemia. It is not advisable to repeatedly perform blood tests to check for anemia in your child. Doing so may actually cause anemia from the recurrent blood sampling.

If significant anemia is present, the child may feel fatigued, experience headaches, or have breathing difficulties. Keep in mind that these symptoms do not manifest themselves until the concentration of red blood cells has fallen to a critically low level. You cannot always rely on these symptoms to detect anemia.

Since fatigue does not occur from anemia until the blood level is extremely low, it is not a common symptom of anemia. If your child experiences significant fatigue, there might be other potentially serious medical problems. Take your child to the doctor if he is unusually tired.

Causes of Anemia

Insufficient dietary intake of iron is by far the most common cause of anemia in children. This is why pediatricians emphasize the importance of a balanced diet. Another important cause of anemia is chronic intestinal bleeding. This is less common in children than adults, but its possibility must be considered when diagnosing and treating anemia. Other causes of anemia include rare inherited blood disorders, such as sickle cell anemia and thalassemia. The other causes are responsible for a very small fraction of anemic children.

Blood Tests for Anemia

Pediatricians regularly screen for anemia during routine well-child visits. The first anemia screen is usually done around one year of age, and once every two years is usually sufficient for healthy children over the age of two.

There are two ways to obtain blood samples when checking for anemia. The finger-prick method is fast and relatively pain-less, but it's not nearly as reliable as the blood sample taken from the vein directly. Doctors take all the factors into consideration when they select one method over the other.

Scheduled Bleeding

Adolescent girls who started menstruating at a young age are at a higher risk for developing anemia than their nonmenstruating peers and boys. Coupled with a less-than-desirable diet of junk foods and irregular eating habits, these young girls are especially susceptible to developing anemia.

If your daughter has heavy menstrual bleeding or frequent spotting, make sure she's eating enough meat and other iron-rich foods. If not, consider checking her for anemia annually.

Strong Teeth

Fluoridation of the public water supply has been one of the favorite topics of conspiracy theorists. It was prominently featured in the film *Doctor Strangelove*, and even professional organizations are constantly changing their official recommendation as far as whether fluoride supplements are needed. This section summarizes the current understanding of the subject matter and dispels the common myths associated with fluoridation.

What Is Fluoride?

Fluoride is a simple substance that naturally occurs in nature. It is not a synthetic chemical. Even without active fluoridation of water, all creatures are exposed to low levels in the environment from natural soil and rocks.

Most people agree that the natural low level of fluoride is completely harmless, but it is also too low to have any beneficial effect in maintaining healthy teeth. The whole controversy started when the first scientific evidence demonstrated that additional fluoride in the diet can help prevent dental cavities.

Cavity Fighter

In the last four decades, dental cavities in children have become less common than they used to be, and many dental experts credit fluoridation of the water supply for this reduction. Numerous sound scientific studies have shown that fluoride has a clear role in preventing dental cavities and even reversing early cavities. What's controversial about fluoride is whether it's harmful and what method is best for incorporating trace amounts of it into the body.

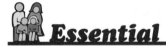 **Essential**

Fluoride protects the teeth in many ways, including strengthening them by making them resistant to erosion from acid. In addition, fluoride also helps the body repair existing tooth decay. These two beneficial effects of fluoride form a potent one-two punch to knock out potential cavities.

The subject of flouridation is made even more confusing by the different standards each local community adopts when it comes to fluoridation of the public water supply. Some cities do not add fluoride to the water at all, while others add a variation of concentrations. There is no consensus, even among experts in public health, as to the optimal level of fluoridation of the public water supply.

Today, there are two major ways that fluoride can be introduced to children. The first method requires fluoride to be applied to the teeth directly. This can either be accomplished by adding fluoride to commercial toothpastes or by dental application during regular visits to the dentist. Certain types of mouth rinse also contain fluoride. The surfaces of the teeth are directly exposed to fluoride in this method.

An alternative is to introduce fluoride to the drinking water, so once the body absorbs the fluoride into the bloodstream, it can be incorporated into children's developing teeth. This method also exposes the surface of the teeth to fluoride because it is present in the saliva once the body absorbs it into the bloodstream.

The Bottom Line

Most pediatricians no longer routinely recommend fluoride supplementation to healthy children. This is especially true because most local communities do supply varying levels of fluoride in the public water source. The additional fluoride supplementation would put young children at risk of getting excessive amounts of fluoride.

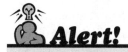

Alert!

Aside from dental discoloration, excessive fluoride does not cause any harm to any other tissue or organ, as far as the medical community is aware. It does not cause any neurological or physical problems, as alleged by antifluoridation activists.

Instead, pediatricians recommend the use of a fluoridated toothpaste in children starting at age two. Make sure you only use a pea-sized amount of toothpaste; otherwise, any toothpaste that is accidentally swallowed can provide your child with too much fluoride. To further limit the total amount of daily fluoride exposure, do not brush your child's teeth more than twice a day.

CHAPTER 17

Bones and Joints

B ones and joints in children are very different from those same parts of the adult body. They actively grow, and even though they are more resilient, they are more prone to special types of injuries not seen in adults. Even the normal task of growing sometimes brings discomfort to children. Parents must be able to distinguish the normal from the pathologic to decide when to seek medical attention for their child's aches and pains.

Accident Waiting

Children are more prone to injuries than adults. They just love to push their physical ability to the limit when they test their boundaries and explore the world around them. Fortunately, their bodies are also blessed with quick recovery and fast healing. The job of parents and pediatricians is only a supportive one, providing comfort and assistance during the healing phase.

Fractures
Fractures of the extremities are common in children, mostly because children are more reckless with their bodies than adults. At the same time, most fractures in children are less serious than in adults because young bones are more pliable; they can bend significantly before breaking.

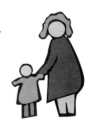

The most common types of fractures involve the wrist and the collarbone. Children love to run around, but the faster they run, the harder they fall when they trip. Climbing also puts these young bones at risk for injuries. Trauma to the limbs is almost routine in children, and parents must decide when to bring their child to the doctor's office.

Almost all fractures require casting, with the exception of fingers and toes. Unless the injury has broken the skin, or circulation of the limb is affected, casting does not need to be done immediately. If your child's fingers or toes feel numb or cold, you have to bring him to the emergency room without delay. Sometimes a fracture can be so severe that the blood supply to the body beyond the injury is disrupted—an absolute surgical emergency.

 Essential

Significant swelling at the site of injury that persists for more than a few hours is likely to be an indication of a fracture. If the area is simply bruised, the swelling and pain usually subside after a few hours. If your child refuses to use the limb due to pain a few hours after an injury, you should consider taking him to the doctor.

Most bones require six to eight weeks to heal completely, and that's the typical duration for a cast before it is removed. During the healing process, the bone specialist may wish to check on the progress of the fracture by taking X-rays through the cast. This is often done if the initial injury is severe.

Sprains and Strains

Sprains and strains are far more common than fractures in children because their bones are not as brittle while their ligaments are very stretchy. The good thing is that sprains and strains heal much more rapidly than fractures, and no rigid support system (such as a cast) is necessary during the healing process.

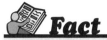 *Fact*

A sprain is an injury to a ligament, which is a tough tissue connecting two bones. A strain is an injury to a muscle or the part of the muscle that attaches to a bone. One condition isn't necessarily more serious than the other—both conditions can range from mild to severe.

The most common place for a sprain is the ankle. If your child's foot lands on an uneven surface, the entire weight of the body forces the foot to roll to the side and twist the ankle joint. This is the most common mechanism for an ankle sprain. Other sprains can occur with a fall or a strong impact. A minor sprain causes some of the microscopic fibers in the tissue to unravel, but a severe sprain can cause a complete disruption of all the fibers in the connective tissue.

Muscle strain typically occurs when a muscle is stretched beyond its maximal length. The opposing muscle may be responsible for the overstretching, but a fall or collision (such as running into another person) is equally likely to cause the overstretching.

Immediate pain always follows a sprain, but the pain with a strain can be somewhat delayed. There may or may not be a bruise on the skin on the surface of the injured site, but function is almost always restricted as a result of the injury.

The mnemonic "RICE" is a good one to keep in mind when treating your child with a sprain or strain. It stands for "rest, ice, compression, and elevate." Allowing enough recovery time for the injury is perhaps the most important aspect of managing a sprain or strain. Parents must remind their child that it requires a tremendous amount of patience and discipline to wait until the injury heals before resuming sports activities. Otherwise, the child is setting himself up for more serious injuries.

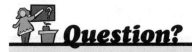 *Question?*

Is an icepack or a heating pad better after an injury?
Using a cold pack is always a good idea for an acute injury. Make sure that the cold surface is not in direct contact with the skin; otherwise, frostbite might occur. Heating pads are generally used for chronic injuries or arthritis, which usually occur in adults.

Recovery from a sprain or strain typically takes two weeks. At the end of the recovery, the child should slowly return to normal activity levels. If any discomfort or pain recurs, the child should stop immediately. This is the body's signal that the injury has not healed completely, and more time must be allowed for the body part to repair itself. Exercising through pain and a partially healed injury is foolish and dangerous.

Proper use of a compression bandage can provide additional support during healing. The additional support is not designed to allow the child to return to athletic activities prematurely but to protect the injured area during routine activities.

Elevating the extremity can reduce swelling and pain. In addition to elevation, taking anti-inflammatory medications, such as ibuprofen, is a good idea to minimize swelling and promote comfort.

Developmental Hip Dysplasia

Developmental hip dysplasia is a condition that affects babies. It used to be called congenital hip dysplasia, but the nomenclature was changed because doctors later realized that this condition is not always present at birth. Congenital implies a condition that occurs prior to birth or right at birth.

Hip dysplasia occurs when the thighbone, or femur, becomes dislocated from the hipbone. Normally, one end of the femur should be connected to a socket of the hipbone. When dislocation occurs, the femur separates from the hipbone. If the joint remains dislocated, permanent deformity may occur to the hip joint, and the child may never walk again.

The Cause

No one is certain about the true causes of hip dysplasia. There are probably several factors that contribute to the condition. Researchers do know that baby girls are more likely to develop hip dysplasia than baby boys, and babies who are born breech (delivered legs first) tend to get hip dysplasia more often. In addition, overcrowding inside the uterus also predisposes babies to hip dysplasia.

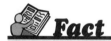 **Fact**

Developmental dysplasia of the hip is a relatively common condition. It is estimated to affect 4 out of 1,000 babies. The risk of having the condition is higher in firstborn babies, and girls are six to nine times more likely to have the condition than boys.

How is hip dysplasia diagnosed? Pediatricians check hip dysplasia in all babies born in the hospital, usually within twenty-four hours of birth. The doctor holds each leg in a hand and pushes down on the hip joint. If hip dysplasia is present, the joint is temporarily dislocated. If the doctor detects hip instability, an ultrasound is ordered to confirm the diagnosis.

Treatment

Luckily, most babies with hip dysplasia can be treated non-surgically. A specially designed strap that roughly resembles a suspender is used to correctly hold the thighbone in the socket of the hipbone. As the baby grows, the correct placement of the bones in the joints encourages proper growth, and dislocation is prevented by the harness. This contraption must be worn at all times, and it must be serially adjusted by a physician. More than 90 percent of babies with hip dysplasia get better with this harness.

If the harness fails to fix the problem, the baby needs to be put in a bulky leg-length cast for many months to allow the bone to develop undisturbed. If that fails, parts of the thighbone may need to be surgically reshaped to fit into the socket of the hipbone. Fortunately, this procedure is rarely necessary.

In and Out

In-toeing and out-toeing are common concerns for parents. In the past, doctors recommended steel leg braces to correct these common conditions, but doctors now know these braces are largely unnecessary. In-toeing and out-toeing are extremely common, and most correct themselves as the child grows.

Walk This Way

Many parents are concerned about their baby's feet because they appear to point outward instead of forward. This is actually a normal finding in most babies, but some deviations are more pronounced than others. The feet appear to point outward because of the crowded condition inside the uterus prior to birth. Once the baby is delivered, the bones gradually straighten out on their own, although it can take quite a while for this to happen.

Pigeon-Toed

Older children are more likely to have in-toeing problem. When this occurs in a baby, the condition is probably the result of crowding inside the uterus. However, when this condition exists in school-age children, it may be caused by either rotation of the lower leg or the thighbone.

Toddlers are more likely to have a slight twisting of their lower leg bones. This is a benign condition that usually normalizes with time. Some older children have a rotated thighbone because of the way they sit. These children are often found to sit on the floor with their legs bent underneath them and outward in the shape of a "W." Habitual sitting in this fashion can cause the hip joint to splay out, which leads to in-toeing.

 Essential

Orthopedic shoes, braces, and cables were once used to correct the gait of children with in-toeing and out-toeing. These contraptions are now proven to be completely ineffective and worthless, despite their popular historic use.

Encourage your child to sit cross-legged on the floor instead of with legs splayed out. This will gradually correct the bony deformity over the course of many months to years. It is extremely rare for these conditions to require surgical intervention.

Nursemaid's Elbow

Nursemaid's elbow is an idyllic name for a not-so-bucolic condition. It is a partial dislocation of the elbow. It mostly affects children under the age of five, but older children may occasionally suffer from it also.

Your child will most likely cry out in pain immediately after the dislocation occurs. After a few minutes he may stop crying but still refuse to use the arm. Most commonly, he will bend his arm at the elbow while the other hand holds the injured arm at the wrist. Since holding of the wrist is a common posture, many parents mistakenly believe that there is an injury at the wrist. Of course, the real location of the pain is at the elbow.

As long as the elbow remains dislocated, your child will not move the arm. The fingers and wrist can move normally, but the toddler usually cannot reach out and grab anything with that arm. This can go on for days if the dislocation is not corrected.

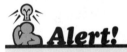

Alert!

If you need to pick up your toddler, never pull her up by the hand or wrist. Put your hands under her armpits or around her waist when lifting her. Many caring parents unwittingly injure their child by lifting the body by the hands, thus dislocating the elbow.

Luckily, this problem has a quick and easy fix. The doctor will first evaluate the arm carefully to ensure that there is no fracture or other injuries. After the doctor feels confident that the diagnosis is nursemaid's elbow, all it takes is a fast bending and rotating of the elbow joint to snap the ligament back to its proper location. This maneuver can trigger some moderate discomfort, but the pain goes away immediately after the elbow joint is fixed.

The arm may regain its function in just a few minutes, or it may take up to a few hours, depending on how long ago the dislocation occurred and how motivated the child is to use the arm. On rare occasions, the dislocation may require more than one attempt to get it fixed. If your child still doesn't use the arm a day after the fix, bring him back to the doctor to get rechecked.

Growing Pains

Even though growing pains do not cause any permanent damage to the bones or joints, they can cause significant amount of discomfort at times.

Limb Pain

Pain in the lower legs is the most common type of growing pain. This type of pain usually occurs at night, as the child is getting ready to go to sleep. The pain can involve just one leg or both legs, and the child frequently asks the parent to rub it or put a warm compress on it. This pain can persist for half an hour or more, but it shouldn't prevent the child from ultimately falling asleep.

The most likely explanation for growing pain is that the bone can sometimes grow at a faster rate than the outer covering of the bone. When this occurs, the covering of the bone is stretched beyond its normal size, and the tension causes pain. It's not unlike having your child dressed in clothes that are two sizes too small. As the bone lengthens, it puts stress on the covering of the bone until it, too, stretches to keep up with the growth.

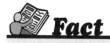 **Fact**

The hallmark for this type of growing pain is that it is always gone by the morning. It seldom occurs on a daily basis, and it rarely prevents the child from running and playing during the day. This pain is part of the normal growing process, so it is not associated with fever or weight loss.

Chest Pain

It is always alarming for a child to complain of a pain in the chest. Luckily, the vast majority of chest pains in children are innocuous. By far, the most common cause for a chest pain in a child is a particular type of growing pain known as costochondritis.

This condition usually occurs at rest although it can also occur during active periods. Similar to the other type of growing pain, the rate of growth of the ribs sometimes outpaces that of the cartilaginous connection of the ribs. This results in elevated tension in the rib connections to the central breastbone.

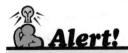

Alert!

If your child has a history of heart problem or asthma, do not hesitate to bring her to the doctor's office when she experiences chest pain. A typical case of costochondritis should not cause dizziness or coughing. Even if the chest pain turns out to be benign, it is better to be safe than sorry.

When evaluating costochondritis, the pediatrician carefully listens to the heart and lungs of your child to rule out other problems that might cause chest pain. In addition, the doctor will probably press her fingers against various spots on the chest to attempt to recreate the painful sensation. If the pain can be reproduced this way, then a diagnosis of costochondritis is confirmed.

Like other types of growing pain, costochondritis resolves on its own once growth is complete. It is likely to come and go as your child grows, so there is no need to fret each time this occurs. The pain can usually be eased with ibuprofen, assuming it lasts for more than a few minutes.

CHAPTER 18

The Importance of Good Sleep

Agood night's sleep is often taken for granted. But for many parents with babies and young children, it's as difficult to attain as the Holy Grail. Sleep problems change as a child develops, and you must understand the facts and misconceptions behind your children's sleep requirement and pattern to better facilitate the quality sleep their young bodies need. In addition, a good night's sleep for your children often means a good night's rest for you.

Normal Sleep Cycles

Sleep is not as passive as it initially appears. In fact, scientists are still uncertain about exactly what happens to the brain when a person is asleep. This downtime may have diverse and essential roles in growth and development, the formation of memory, the acquisition of new skills, or the process of the brain "downsizing" itself by getting rid of unnecessary connections between nerves. However, one thing is certain: Without quality sleep, nobody can function effectively for very long.

Stages of Sleep

There are two general types of sleep—the one involved with dreaming and the other without. The type of sleep that occurs while dreaming is described as REM (rapid eye movement) sleep, and

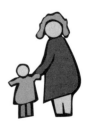

the other is called non-REM sleep. REM sleep is named because during this type of sleep, the eyes dart rapidly back and forth, even though the eyelids are shut. Dreams occur during this type of sleep, and the brain is almost as active as it is in waking states. During non-REM sleep, the brain is calm. Ironically, it is during non-REM sleep when many of the problems associated with sleep, such as bed-wetting and sleepwalking, occur.

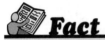 **Fact**

It is true that everyone wakes up several times a night, including adults. Most adults don't even open their eyes during these transition periods. They simply shift their body's position slightly and fall right back to sleep. Babies, on the other hand, sometimes have a much harder time falling back to sleep on their own.

Throughout the night, the brain goes through many cycles of REM and non-REM sleep, alternating between the two types. For infants, the cycles rotate much faster, in approximately sixty-minute intervals. As the child grows older, the cycles slow down, turning over every ninety minutes or so. It is during this transition from REM to non-REM sleep that a baby is most likely to wake up. Due to the shorter cycles, infants wake up more often at night than older children.

How Much Sleep Is Enough?

The total number of hours of sleep varies depending on the age of the child and individual differences. Just as body size and appetite differ significantly from one person to the next, the requirement for sleep also varies widely. While there is no absolute "right" amount of sleep for everyone, there are general patterns for different age groups.

It is obvious that babies generally require more sleep than older children. Newborns typically go through short two- to three-hour cycles of feeding, playing, and sleeping throughout the day. Their sleep pattern is not dictated by the sunlight at all but rather by their internal rhythm. If you add up all the hours of naps, an average newborn sleeps about fifteen to eighteen hours in a twenty-four-hour period.

As your baby becomes older, the total amount of sleep decreases, and the sleep cycle becomes more in tune with a circadian rhythm (that is, the pattern established by sunlight). By six months, most babies spend most of the night sleeping and spend longer periods of time awake during the daytime. Frequent daytime naps are essential to provide enough sleep for these babies.

By the time your child is a toddler (one to three years of age), he needs even less sleep and spends the majority of the day awake and active. Children of this age typically require twelve to fourteen hours of sleep in a twenty-four-hour period. Many of them only nap once or twice a day, spending about an hour or two asleep for each nap.

Once again, it is important to remember that there is a lot of individual variability when it comes to sleep. Many parents worry that there might be something wrong with their child because their toddler does not take naps during the day at all. As long as the child appears well rested and alert during the day and gets quality sleep time at night, there is no need to be concerned about sleep deprivation.

As your child enters adolescence, the requirement for sleep is more similar to that of an adult. However, nine to ten hours of sleep is typically necessary to ensure that your teenager is refreshed in the morning and alert enough to take on the academic tasks at school. Unfortunately, as your teenager becomes more independent, it becomes more difficult to regulate bedtime and the daytime schedule. According to many studies, most adolescents spend their days sleep-deprived—just like most adults.

How can you be sure that your child is sleeping enough? As a good rule of thumb, if your child does not wake up cranky and does not doze off during times when he is expected to be awake, he is getting enough sleep at night.

Sleeping Like a Baby

"Sleeping like a baby" is perhaps one of the cruelest sayings for parents to hear. Most new parents soon realize that many babies do not sleep soundly, and many of them can fuss for hours before falling to sleep. Some babies get cranky before and after sleeping. In fact, sleep problems are among the most common topics parents ask about during office visits to the pediatrician. If the infant has problems with sleeping, the parents are more likely to be sleep-deprived as well, and this can interfere with the bonding process between parents and baby. Left unresolved, sleep problems can become a serious crisis for the entire family.

Establishing a Routine

Having strict feeding time, play time, and naptime is paramount in establishing a regular schedule for your baby. When your baby first wakes up, she is most likely going to be hungry. Satisfying her hunger is the most logical next step. After she is satiated, she is usually alert for a brief period of time. This is the time when your baby is most interested in playing. After she becomes exhausted from playing, she will be ready for her next nap again. This sequence of feeding, playing, and napping is the most fundamental component of a baby's routine.

This said, each baby usually has some personal quirks in her routine. Look for feedback from your baby and learn from her. Do not go against her preference in the routine. If the baby appears tired after feeding, don't force her to play with you. If the baby wants to play for a long period of time after feeding, don't force her to go to sleep. Find out what your baby wants, and go with the flow. Know the fundamentals of establishing routines, but be flexible at the same time. Respecting these idiosyncrasies will make both baby and parents happier.

Essential

Just like adults, most babies appreciate routines. Routines allow them to expect when they are going to be fed, when they play, and when they take naps. Babies with a well-established schedule thrive on it, and they are generally happier. When babies are happy, the parents are more likely to be happy, too.

Training Your Baby to Sleep

Falling asleep is a learned skill. It does not come naturally for most babies. The idea of teaching your baby how to fall asleep should not sound like such a strange idea. In fact, it is one of the first skills your child has to master. This milestone can be accomplished quickly, or it can become a long drawn-out battle between you and your baby. The following discussion will guide you through the process relatively pain-free.

During the transition between REM and non-REM sleep, all babies go through a stage of relative light sleep. Many of them wake up. It is during this time that they must figure out how to fall back to sleep on their own. If they do not know how to do so, they will start fussing and wake up crying.

When your baby wakes up in the middle of the night and starts fussing, this is the perfect opportunity for you to start teaching your baby how to fall back to sleep unassisted. Pediatricians recommend training your baby gradually. The first time your baby cries, check on him to make sure that nothing is making him uncomfortable. Ensure that he's not stuck in an uncomfortable position, the room temperature is not too hot or too cold, and his diaper is not soiled. If everything looks fine, try not to pick him up and hold him. Allow him to fuss for five to ten minutes before picking him up and soothing him back to sleep. Picking him up immediately at the first sign of fussiness deprives him of the opportunity to learn how to soothe himself back to sleep. Keep in mind that this approach does not apply to infants less than two months old.

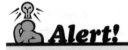

Alert!

A common myth is that you should rock the baby in your arms until she has fallen asleep, and then put her to bed. This method often causes the baby to wake up immediately after you lay her in the crib, and crying frequently begins. The trick is to put the baby to bed before she is asleep but after she is already drowsy.

While you do want your baby to gradually learn how to return to sleep on her own, you don't want her to cry all night either. First of all, it is extremely difficult for parents to hear their baby cry without doing something to stop the crying. Some parents may find it impossible to hold off on picking their baby up once the crying starts. It's no doubt a tough thing to ask of parents, but if the baby does not learn how to self-soothe, he will keep waking up at night and requiring his parents to put him back to sleep until he's a toddler. Many schoolchildren still need their parents to coax them back to bed when they wake up at night. Sooner or later, they have to master this skill. It is usually a good thing to do so earlier, for the sake of the child and the parents.

Introducing Solids Early

Many parents believe that by introducing solids earlier to their babies, especially at night, they can better fill up the baby and allow the baby to sleep longer at night. This myth ranks among the most popular and most entrenched old wives' tales in all of pediatrics. Not only is this practice ineffective, it may even harm your baby.

Pediatricians and dieticians recommend postponing the introduction of solids until the baby is at least six months old. This means that prior to that age, the infant should feed on either breast milk or commercial infant formula. Absolutely nothing else should be fed to the baby.

This recommendation is made based on the observation that babies who start on solids earlier than six months tend to develop more food-related allergies in childhood and adulthood. In addition, babies lack the necessary motor skills and neck muscle support for ingesting solids. Introducing baby cereal too early increases the risk of choking.

Sudden Infant Death Syndrome (SIDS)

One of the greatest discoveries in pediatrics in the past century was the realization that by putting babies on their backs to sleep, parents can dramatically decrease the chance of their baby dying from sudden infant death syndrome (SIDS). This single piece of advice has saved more lives than any other recommendation made by pediatricians in modern medical history.

Before embarking on a detailed discussion about this practice, it is important to clarify the definition of SIDS. SIDS is when babies less than one year old who are completely healthy die in their sleep for no apparent reason. Even though SIDS can occur to any baby less than twelve months of age, it is most common in babies less than six months old. It happens to approximately one in every thousand babies. There are minimal autopsy findings from infants who have died from SIDS, and these find-ings are not very enlightening in revealing the cause of death.

Back to Sleep

From expert consensus on the topic, SIDS is most likely caused by rebreathing a small pocket of air. For some reason yet to be identified, some babies seem to be unable to turn their heads or shuffle their posture when they are sleeping. Usually, this doesn't pose any specific threat, unless the baby is lying face down and is repeatedly breathing a small pocket of air around the face. Over an extended period of time, the oxygen level in this small pocket is depleted and the carbon dioxide level builds up from exhaled air. It is hypothesized that this stale air ultimately suffocates the baby by depriving the baby's brain of oxygen.

 Essential

Since 1992, the American Academy of Pediatrics has recommended that all babies under the age of one year be placed on their backs when they sleep. Since the announcement of this guideline, the number of babies dying from SIDS has dropped by more than 40 percent. There is no question that this single recommendation has made the biggest impact in the reduction of SIDS.

Assuming this explanation is the real cause of SIDS, it does make intuitive sense that by placing babies on their back, this rebreathing of air can largely be prevented. Nevertheless, there are still babies dying from SIDS despite the widespread use of this practice. This fact suggests that there is probably more than one cause of SIDS, and scientists have not yet identified all of them.

There are other risk factors associated with SIDS, including maternal smoking, soft bedding, the presence of toys in the crib, and cosleeping. As additional risk factors are being elucidated, some of these new findings are controversial. In all likelihood, SIDS has multiple causes. The propensity for SIDS is probably determined somewhat by genetics, but various other environmental factors can increase the risk for SIDS. Until the scientists can ascertain all the possible causes for SIDS, pediatricians recommend curbing all of these additional risk factors.

Cosleeping with Adults

This is among the most controversial topics in pediatrics. Recent studies have shown that the incidence of SIDS is higher for babies who sleep in the same bed with adults. It appears that the risk is particularly high when the adult involved is excessively drowsy, intoxicated, or is a smoker. The reason for this observation is not entirely clear, but it may have something to do with an overly sedated adult rolling over on top of the infant or accidentally turning the baby onto her stomach.

The evidence against cosleeping is pretty solid, but many parents insist on doing so because of cultural practices. To strike a compromise, you can pull the crib close to your bed, so the baby is still nearby but does not share the same bed with any adults. If you absolutely must sleep with your baby in the same bed, make sure that you do not consume alcohol or smoke during the day. You should not take any medication that might cause you to be excessively drowsy. Once again, a growing number of pediatricians strongly discourage parents from cosleeping with their infants under any circumstances.

Sleeping on the Side

Putting babies on their sides to sleep has been a controversial topic, but it shouldn't be. Clinical studies have proven beyond any doubt that by placing babies on their sides, the risk of SIDS is significantly higher than if they are put on their backs. The vast majority of healthy infants should never be put to bed on their sides. This practice should not be condoned, despite what some parental or medical organizations claim.

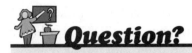

Question?

What should I do if my baby rolls onto her stomach, instead of lying on her back?
There is no reason to be alarmed. By the time the baby is coordinated and strong enough to roll over to her stomach on her own, she is more than likely able to shift her position when she is sleeping and avoid rebreathing the same stale air.

Some parents still allow their babies to sleep on their side because they fear that their babies might choke when they spit up if they're sleeping on their back. However, this concern has never been validated by any scientific studies. No healthy baby has ever been reported to choke to death because of spitting up during sleep. The main explanation for this is that the neurological system of a baby is actually quite advanced when it comes to protecting the lungs from being flooded with milk or saliva. Since such a reflex is crucial for survival, this sophisticated system is firmly in place by the time a full-term infant is born. Some premature babies and babies with serious neurological problems might not have this reflex intact, and these are the rare exceptions when parents should place their babies to sleep on their sides. Ask your doctor whether you should do so if you are unsure.

Nightmares and Night Terrors

To watch a child wake up screaming can induce a lot of stress in a parent. Whether the behavior is triggered by the child's memory of a frightful dream or night terror, the experience is just as terrifying for the parents. The good news is that these conditions are benign and do not cause any psychological harm to the child. Knowing why they happen and what to do can also minimize the psychological damage to parents.

Beware of the Dark Side

Many toddlers resist going to bed on their own because they are afraid of the dark. Even though this is typically the age when they start to assert their independence, this is also the age when they start to develop a fanciful imagination. All sorts of demons and monsters may haunt their creative minds, especially once the lights go out.

You can remedy the situation by leaving a night light on. Avoid watching scary television programs or movies before going to bed. Spend the time after dinner quietly doing some relaxing and nonstimulating activities. If it helps your child to go through the entire room checking for monsters, you can incorporate the ritual as a part of the bedtime routine. Reassure your child that there is no monster under the bed or in the closet. It is generally not worth the time to reason with a toddler that there is no such thing as a monster or boogie man. Going through a long discussion about these scary things may further heighten the anxiety of your toddler.

Night Terrors

Night terrors are not as familiar to parents as nightmares, and these two conditions are completely different and unrelated. Even though your child may react similarly to them, what you should do for your child when she has an episode of night terror is very different from what you would for a nightmare.

Night terrors occur at a stage of deep sleep. Your child is not fully conscious during these episodes. Typically what happens during night terror is that your child starts screaming at the top of her lungs in the middle of the night. This usually happens several hours after she has fallen asleep. She stares blankly into space and does not respond to you. It can be very disconcerting for parents to witness such an event.

The best thing to do is to lay your child back down and pat her to calm her down. It is not a good idea to wake her up. Stay with her until the screaming stops. She'll usually fall back to sleep spontaneously. Unfortunately, this can take anywhere from a few minutes to more than an hour. The most important thing to keep in mind is that this condition is harmless, despite its frightening appearance. Your child will not remember any incident of night terror the following morning. There is no need to bring up the subject and force your child to remember anything that happened the night before.

Insomnia

Insomnia does not only affect adults, as millions of children also suffer from it from time to time. However, insomnia in children is more likely to have an easier solution. For one thing, children's lives tend to be less complicated and stressful than those of adults. Furthermore, their sleep cycle is less likely to be influenced by alcohol or caffeine. There are several good pieces of advice to keep in mind to help your child fall asleep.

Causes of Sleeplessness in Children

While insomnia is an extremely common problem in adults, it tends to affect only older children. Fortunately, the etiology of pediatric insomnia is generally easier to identify. The most common trigger for sleeplessness in children is stress.

As your child grows older, her social life becomes more complex. Academics, friends, sports, and even family members can all be sources of stress for a child. Unresolved tension during the day can intrude into the night and interfere with sleep.

Besides a television, many children have their own computers in the bedroom. When the temptation of a live online community is right there, the urge to chat with friends into the wee hours of the morning or play online games until dawn can be too much for many children to resist.

What You Can Do

First and foremost, it is important to establish a regular bed-time for your child. The human body obeys a circadian rhythm that helps people regulate a sleep-wake cycle. Once firmly in place, this cycle can help you fall asleep faster and easier. Unfortunately, many adolescents have the habit of staying up late and waking up late during the weekends, thereby breaking this cycle. Once Monday comes along, they have to readjust to the old schedule. Encourage your child to stick with the same schedule during the weekends. This solution will go a long way toward curbing your child's insomnia problem.

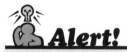

Alert!

Beside stress, distractions in the bedroom are a major cause of insomnia in children. Television in the bedroom isn't a good idea for maintaining a healthy weight for your child, and it isn't a good thing for falling asleep either. Falling asleep with the television set on is terrible for the establishment of a good sleeping habit.

While you cannot make your child fall asleep, you can make her stay awake during the times when she should be awake. Try not letting her sleep in or take naps, even if her schedule allows such downtime. You might be doing her a favor. Sleeping during the time when she should not be sleeping could only make falling asleep more difficult at bedtime.

Try your best to address the specific stresses in your child's life. While some sources of stress are beyond your control, it is nevertheless important to discuss them with your child. Children might have an exaggerated fear of a situation and worry excessively about something that may not be as threatening as they perceive.

Remove any potential distractions from the bedroom. Video games or television should not be kept in your child's bedroom. In addition, restrict the hours your child spends online.

Finally, parents should limit children's caffeine intake during the day. Caffeinated beverages can wreak havoc on the sleep pattern and potentially cause academic difficulties and trigger safety concerns.

Some children take medications that might interfere with their sleep cycle. If the medication is disrupting sleep, talk to your doctor about the possibility of adjusting the timing and dosage of the medication. Usually, an alternative way of dosing the medication can be used to avert this problem.

A Cautionary Tale of Sedative

Aiding your child's sleep with sedatives should be considered only as a method of last resort. If you do choose to use a sedative, do so only on a short-term basis. Many medications have a high potential for abuse and addiction. Beside, it is more important to identify the underlying cause of insomnia in your child than to simply cover it up with sedatives.

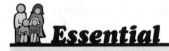 **Essential**

If you want to consider something natural to help your child fall asleep, try a glass of milk prior to bedtime. Milk contains the amino acid tryptophan, which is converted into serotonin and melatonin once it is absorbed in the body. Both of these chemicals having soporific properties, and they have been shown to induce sleep in clinical studies.

Most pediatricians agree that the only appropriate role for sedatives in alleviating children's insomnia is during periods of high stress. For example, sedatives can be safely used in the days leading up to a major elective surgery or during hospitalization. Once the stress resolves, the sedative should be discontinued immediately to curb any potential for dependence.

Chapter 19

Infection Control Runs Amuck

From an infectious disease's standpoint, day cares and schools are nothing more than a stock exchange for germs. School and public officials are to be lauded for their efforts in preventing outbreaks of illnesses in this public setting, but sometimes their well-intentioned strategy backfires. This is especially likely to happen when policies are made without consideration of sound scientific facts.

Of Lice and Men

Head lice have been around for thousands of years. They have even been found in prehistoric mummies. This insect lives exclusively on the human head, so it's impossible to catch head lice from animals. Contrary to common belief, this condition can occur in children of any socioeconomic levels. No child is immune.

Lousy Transmission

Head lice are transmitted primarily by direct head-to-head contact, but it is possible to catch head lice by using other people's combs or sharing hats. Lice are actually not as contagious as most people believe. These bugs cannot jump or fly, so they are virtually impossible to catch without direct physical contact.

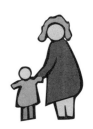

The Exterminator

Before initiation of treatment, make sure you have the correct diagnosis. Without an accurate diagnosis, you cannot expect to see a resolution of the problem. Frequently, other problems such as dandruff or skin conditions such as psoriasis are the cause of an itchy scalp.

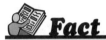 **Fact**

The "no-nit" policy of many schools is completely groundless. As long as there are no live lice around, the child is not infectious. Long after the successful eradication of head lice, most children will still retain hundreds of dead louse eggs in their hair. These children should not be prevented from attending school.

Over-the-counter louse-killing shampoos are usually quite effective in getting rid of an infestation. Follow the instructions on these medications carefully, and do not use them excessively without the supervision of medical personnel.

Remember, treatment is only necessary when the presence of a live louse has been detected and confirmed. Dead egg sacs do not pose any problem, and repeated treatment is futile.

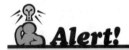 **Alert!**

Many folk remedies for head lice are potentially dangerous. Some people have tried lighting matches to burn off the nits, or using toxic or caustic chemicals to burn the lice off. These measures are more likely to cause serious harm to your child than the lice you're targeting.

If you are concerned about contaminated personal items that might harbor lice, you can store objects such as pillowcases, pajamas, hats, or combs in a large, sealed, airtight trash bag for a week. Any live lice or viable eggs present will hatch during this time, and the new lice will starve to death.

Adult lice feed on human blood. They cannot survive for more than a day without feeding. This means that if a louse falls off a child's head and cannot find a new head to claim, it will starve to death fairly quickly.

Radioactive Green Mucus

Once a child's mucus turns green, it automatically becomes "radioactive" in the eyes of a day-care provider. However, this change in color and consistency of mucus is often a sign of recovery. The amount of mucus decreases as a child recovers from a cold or flu. The reduction in the volume of mucus in effect thickens it. The green color comes from the dead immune cells that fought the infection.

In general, children suffering from minor colds do not need to be kept home from school. The exception for this rule is during the winter flu season. Unlike the viruses that cause the common cold, the flu virus is extremely contagious. It is easily communicable by air, and if you believe your child has the flu, it is a good idea to keep him home until he recovers. Nevertheless, most children with the flu become contagious a day prior to becoming ill, so school outbreaks of the flu are virtually inevitable.

It does make sense to teach your child to cover her mouth when she coughs or sneezes. This is a simple control measure, but it can make quite an impact. It's also easy enough to learn, even for children less than ten years old. Just remind your child to wash her hands after coughing or sneezing into them. Otherwise, the hands become the perfect vehicle for transporting germs to the next victim.

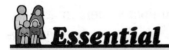
Essential

While some infections can indeed pass from one child to the next via airborne droplets, the vast majority of infections, including the common cold, are transmitted by touch. If children can be made to wash their hands frequently when they are sick, most infectious transmission can be prevented.

Infection control in the school setting can be tricky, but the risk of infecting other students in the class appears to be a small price to pay for the gain in valuable educational opportunity. Certainly green mucus is not a good reason by itself to keep away from other students. Children suffering from chronic allergy miss countless number of days of school due to their constant nasal discharge.

Pink Eye and You

Pink eye is another common childhood malady that causes school administrators to panic. Despite its common occurrence, the eye infection is fortunately relatively harmless in most cases.

What most people mean when they say their child has pink eye is that their child has an infection of the membrane covering the eyeball. However, not all pink-appearing eyes are caused by infections. Even if the redness (or pinkness) is caused by an infection, not all of them get better with antibiotics, because some eye infections are causes by viruses.

Confounding Allergy

Clinicians' first diagnostic priority when they encounter a patient with red eyes is to differentiate an eye infection from an eye allergy. With an eye infection, the redness usually starts abruptly, and it is often accompanied by copious eye discharge and pain. The eye discharge may be so thick and tenacious that your child cannot open his eyes in the morning.

With eye allergy, the onset of symptoms tends to be more insidious. The child may have been bothered by the eye on and off for more than a week, and the eye discharge is usually scant and more watery. Bright light can be bothersome, and irritation with itchiness of the eye is a prominent symptom. Both eyes are often affected together, even though it is possible for an allergic reaction to occur in just one eye.

The physician may question you in order to distinguish an eye infection from an allergic reaction. The treatment is completely different, so it's important to determine the exact cause of the redness. Treating an allergic reaction of the eye with antibiotic eye drops is not only futile, the symptoms may even worsen.

Reaction to Eye Drops

Sometimes the antibiotic eye drops prescribed to treat the eye infection can cause the eyes to become even redder. These patients may have an allergic reaction to the antibiotic eye drop. The most common culprit is sulfa eye drops. Make sure your child does not get sulfa-containing eye drops if she is allergic to sulfa drugs.

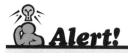

Alert!

If your child wears contact lenses, it is critical that she stop wearing them if she has an eye infection. Reusing contaminated contact lenses causes the child to reinfect herself repeatedly. Do not allow your child to wear disposable contact lenses for prolonged period of time. Follow the recommended replacement schedule.

If your child's pink eye worsens or does not improve after two days of treatment, contact your pediatrician immediately. Look for the word "sulfacetamide" on the label of the eye drops you are using. If you find this word, it means your child is getting a sulfa-containing antibiotic. This antibiotic works well for most eye infections, but if your child is allergic to it, the doctor will have to prescribe an alternate antibiotic for treating pink eye.

Something getting stuck between the eyelids can also cause irritation to the eye and trigger redness. If the doctor suspects this, she may try to wash the eye with a clean liquid to get rid of the foreign body in the eye. In addition, a small cut on the surface of the eye can cause a lot of pain, though it usually does not cause significant discharge.

Back to School

While it is possible to distinguish between an allergic eye reaction and an eye infection, it is virtually impossible to confidently differentiate an eye infection that is caused by virus and one that is caused by bacteria. Consequently, if your pediatrician suspects an eye infection, he is most likely going to treat it with an antibiotic eye drop, even though antibiotics can only cure a bacterial infection.

 Essential

Even though most eye infections get better on their own, it is still worth bringing your child to the doctor to get an infection treated. With treatment, a bacterial eye infection will stop being contagious within twenty-four hours after the initiation of antibiotic eye drops. This may allow your child to return to school sooner.

Regardless of the cause of your child's pink eye, be sure to get a doctor's note after your visit. Without an official release note to return to school, the school administrator may not allow your child to go back to class.

Clean Hands

The effectiveness and importance of hand washing in infection control cannot be overstated. This relatively simple measure is vastly underutilized and underappreciated by the general public. It does not employ the latest health-care technology or any groundbreaking new research, but it is more effective at preventing the spread of infection than any other activity.

Antibacterial Soaps

Antibacterial soap is really an industry gimmick that tricks consumers into spending money unnecessarily. It's based on the popular misconception that antibiotics are the cure-all for all illnesses.

A thorough cleansing using regular soap is just as effective at removing dirt and bacteria from the hands as a wash using antibacterial soap. No scientific study has ever demonstrated any advantage of using antibacterial soaps. Don't waste your money on them.

Waterless Hand Cleansers

These types of alcohol-based hand cleansers have become popular in recent years, and the general consensus in the scientific and medical community is that these are quite effective in preventing the transmission of germs. In fact, this is the rationale behind the practice of wiping down the skin with an alcohol swab prior to injections.

An alcohol-based hand sanitizer is an acceptable alternative to washing the hands with regular soap and water. Waterless sanitizer is especially useful in situations where a running water source is unavailable. Even though these cleansers are very effective in killing germs on the surface of the hands, they are not optimal for removing grease or other stains. For these occasions, regular soap and water is still the way to go.

Proper Hand-Washing Technique

Even when hand washing is appropriately employed as an infection control measure, it is often done incorrectly. The most important aspect of hand washing is not to use generous amounts of soap. The secret lies in the vigorous and meticulous scrubbing. Every surface of the hands must be scrubbed in order to achieve maximum cleanliness.

The human hand has a complex geometry. It has all sorts of nooks and crannies that allow incredible dexterity, yet this very same shape makes thorough cleaning challenging. The trick in washing the entire surface of the hands is to treat each finger and the whole hand as having four sides. In addition, the fingers have an additional side—the tips. To clean each side, you must enthusiastically scrub it back and forth at least five times.

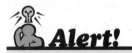

Alert!

In a perfect world, your toddler would stand completely still while you washed her hands, but that's seldom the case. Do your best to thoroughly clean the hands of your squirming child. It may be tempting to hastily wet the hands under running water and call it a day, but doing so risks getting your child and yourself sick.

Start with the thumb, scrub each of the four sides, and proceed to the index finger. Work your way across until you have scrubbed all fingers of both hands. After that, scrub the fingertips.

Finally, scrub the four sides of the entire hand, treating it as a rectangular block. If you follow these instructions correctly, it should take approximately thirty seconds to wash one hand, so it should take almost an entire minute to thoroughly clean both hands.

Cutting corners and performing a cursory hand wash risks missing a part of the hands, and this little crevice may just be the haven for the next virulent strain of drug-resistant bacteria. Keep this possibility in mind every time you wash your hands, and your children's hands, and you'll automatically be a conscientious hand washer.

Public Toilets

Even though many public bathrooms are immaculately cleaned, most parents still fear that letting their child use a public bathroom increases risk of infection. Undoubtedly, some bathrooms are filthy, and the prospect of using them can trigger all sorts of unpleasant responses and disgust. The good news is that it's quite unlikely for anyone to contract an infection simply by sitting on the toilet itself. With proper hand washing and good hygiene practices, using a public toilet can be as safe as eating out in a public restaurant.

Fecal Matter

While the smell of human feces is inherently unpleasant, stools from a healthy individual actually do not pose any health hazard to others. Only when a person becomes ill with a gastrointestinal infection does the stool become contagious.

Of course, no one would advocate not washing hands after going to the bathroom, but an occasional fecal contamination of the hands can be readily remedied by a thorough hand wash. If you or your child happens to touch the toilet or even the feces itself, it's not the end of the world. There's nothing that a careful hand washing cannot fix.

Catching the Cooties

People frequently believe that it's possible to catch infectious diseases by sitting directly on the toilet seat in a public bathroom. This is extremely unlikely.

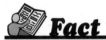 **Fact**

> You cannot catch a sexually transmitted disease (STD) from sitting on a public toilet. All STDs require intimate and prolonged skin-to-skin contact and/or the exchange of bodily fluid. No such thing can occur between your child and the porcelain or plastic surface of the toilet. As long as you wash your child's hands after he uses the toilet, you should both be fine.

From an infectious disease perspective, it is perfectly acceptable to sit your child directly on the toilets in public restrooms. However, if you have any personal objection to having your child's skin touch the toilet seat, don't hesitate to use barrier devices. Keep in mind that you should worry even more when your child insists on opening the door in public places or on pressing the elevator buttons. It's a lot more likely for your child to get germs on the hands than the buttocks.

Appendix A

Glossary

AAP

American Academy of Pediatrics, the official organization for all licensed pediatricians in the United States. It makes official recommendations for pediatricians and parents on how to take care of children in sickness and in health.

ADHD (or ADD)

Attention deficit hyperactivity disorder. A condition in which the affected individual cannot focus attention on a single task for a prolonged period of time.

albuterol

A medication used to treat asthma. It works fast by relaxing the muscles inside the lungs.

allergen

Anything that can trigger an allergic reaction in an individual.

AMA

American Medical Association, the official organization for all licensed physicians in the United States.

anal fissure

A tear to the skin around the anus, caused by passing a stool that stretches the skin a little too much.

anaphylaxis

A severe allergic reaction that involves the entire body. It causes widespread swelling and can potentially be fatal.

anemia

A condition in which the concentration of red blood cells in the body is low.

antihistamines

A group of medications that are typically used to alleviate symptoms of allergy.

asthma

An inflammatory condition affecting the lungs. Common symptoms include chronic nighttime coughing or coughing during exercise.

autism

A neurological condition characterized by the inability to engage in normal social interactions.

baby walker
An extremely dangerous contraption that can cause serious bodily harm to your child.

Benadryl
A common brand-name antihistamine medication used to relieve allergic symptoms. The generic version is called diphenhydramine.

benzoyl peroxide
A popular initial treatment for mild acne (pimples).

BMI
Body mass index, a calculated ratio between weight and height. It helps health professionals in determining whether your child is underweight or overweight.

BRAT
Bananas, rice, apple sauce, and toast. This is the old-school dietary recommendation for treating diarrhea. This is no longer recommended by pediatricians.

bronchiolitis
A viral infection of the lungs that causes wheezing, which can mimic an asthma attack.

CDC
Centers for Disease Control (and Prevention), the principal U.S. government agency for protecting the health and safety of all Americans and for providing essential human services.

colic
Excessive crying in babies for no apparent reason. It is crying that is not the result of any medical problem, pain, gas, or constipation.

corneal abrasion
When the surface of the eye is scratched by a hard object. This can be a very painful condition.

costochondritis
A type of growing pain in children. It's often described as a sudden, sharp pain in the chest.

cryotherapy
When doctors use extreme cold to induce localized frostbite on the skin and destroy warts.

DDAVP
A medication used to manage bedwetting.

dehydration
Excessive loss of bodily fluid, either due to inadequate fluid intake or continual fluid loss from vomiting or diarrhea.

developmental hip dysplasia
An orthopedic condition in which the thighbone becomes dislocated from the hipbone.

DTaP
Diptheria, tetanus, acellular pertussis vaccine, a combination that protects children from serious illness.

dyslexia
A disorder in which symbol recognition and reading comprehension are impaired.

eczema
A term used for chronic skin allergy, although the proper medical terminology for this condition is "atopic dermatitis."

Eustachian tube

A small tube that connects the middle ear and the throat. It helps equalize the pressure between the space inside the middle ear and the outside environment. A plugged Eustachian tube can trigger an ear infection.

FDA

U.S. Food and Drug Administration, the U.S. government agency that monitors drug and food safety in the United States.

fluoride

A chemical that is commonly added to the public water supply to protect teeth from cavities.

folic acid

A type of vitamin B. It is an important supplement that prevents birth defects.

granulation tissue

During the process of healing, this yellowish sticky substance appears on the wound.

hair tourniquet

When a strand of hair wraps itself tightly around a finger, a toe, or even the penis of a very young child. This can cause excruciating pain to the child.

hepatitis

Irritation of the liver by an infection or a chemical.

hydrogen peroxide

A colorless and odorless liquid that destroys healthy tissue. It is no longer recommended to clean cuts and wounds with this chemical.

jaundice

Accumulation of a yellow pigment in the body. This is most commonly seen in newborns. Extremely high levels of the pigment can cause hearing loss and brain damage.

ligament

A tough and fibrous structure that connects bones together. An injury to a ligament is called a sprain.

MMR

Measles, mumps, rubella. A combination childhood vaccine that protects your child from these diseases.

molluscum

A contagious variant of the typical wart.

mucus

A semi-medical term for snot or a wet booger.

non-REM

Deep stages of sleep where dreaming does not occur and the individual is difficult to arouse.

nursemaid's elbow

Partial dislocation of the elbow, a condition that mostly affects children under the age of five.

pneumococcus

A bacterium that is the most common cause of bacterial ear infections and pneumonia in children.

polio

A once-common infection that can cause paralysis and death. Widespread childhood immunization has wiped out this disease in the United States.

pyloric stenosis
A condition in which a baby's stomach muscle is too tight, preventing food from passing through the stomach into the intestines. The baby usually has projectile vomiting.

reflux
Regurgitation of food from the stomach back into the mouth or out.

REM
Rapid eye movement, the stage of sleep where dreaming occurs.

Rubella
Commonly known as German measles. If a pregnant woman contracts this infection, the illness can cause birth defects. Vaccination is the only way to prevent this infection.

scabies
A parasitic infection caused by an eight-legged bug. This skin infestation causes intense itching.

SIDS
Sudden infant death syndrome. It describes the situation in which healthy babies less than one year old die in their sleep for no apparent reason.

spacer
A plastic tube that is connected to an asthma inhaler. This device helps the asthma medication penetrate deep into the lungs. It is expensive and not a disposable device.

sprain
An injury to a ligament, which is a tough tissue connecting two bones.

strain
An injury to a muscle or the part of the muscle that attaches to a bone.

swimmer's ear
An external ear infection that is caused by residual moisture in the ear after swimming or showering.

tetanus
An infection that is contracted by wound contamination. It is usually fatal once the infection is established. Vaccination is the only way to protect your child from this infection.

umbilicus
Medical term for the bellybutton.

whooping cough (pertussis)
A life-threatening infection that can strike people of all ages. Childhood immunization is the only protection against this dangerous infection.

Authoritative Internet Resources

E ven though the Internet provides numerous resources for information about your child's health, it's difficult for busy parents to differentiate the trustworthy from the questionable. You need a reliable source prepared by an expert in the field, using the latest data in academic journals to back up the facts. This section includes authoritative Web sites you can use to find more information on the childhood illnesses addressed in this book.

State Medical Boards
Click on the state you are interested in and proceed to the "find doctor" section of the site. Even though this is a great resource, it only provides a basic background check on your doctor. It does not hint whether the doctor is dedicated to her patients or has a sense of humor. To get beyond fundamentals, you will have to rely on word of mouth.
www.ama-assn.org/ama/pub/category/2645.html

Interesting and Informative Facts on Common Medical Myths

Detailed Discussion on Medical Myths from Aetna InteliHealth
www.intelihealth.com/IH/ihtIH/WSS/9273/35323.html

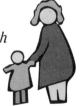

Information on Childhood Obesity

Body Mass Index: Definition and Calculation from the CDC
✐ *www.cdc.gov/nccdphp/ dnpa/bmi/childrens_BMI/ about_childrens_BMI.htm*

Healthy Eating Habits from the American Dietetic Association
✐ *www.wellpoint.com/ healthy_parenting/index.html*

Healthy Living Resources from the Center for Weight and Health, provided by the University of California at Berkeley
✐ *www.cnr.berkeley.edu/cwh/ activities/child_weight2.shtml*

Resources for Colic

Facts about Colic from the Mayo Clinics
✐ *www.mayoclinic.com/health/ colic/DS00058*

Child's Sleep Guide

Resources to Help Solve Your Child's Sleep Problem from the University of Michigan Health System
✐ *www.med.umich.edu/1libr/ yourchild/sleep.htm#baby*

Practical Tips from the National Sleep Foundation
✐ *www.sleepfoundation.org*

Resources on Stuttering

Internet resource
✐ *www.stutteringhelp.org*

Information on Stuttering from the NIH
✐ *www.nidcd.nih.gov/ health/voice/stutter.asp*

What's New on Your Child's Allergy

The journal article on pets and development of childhood allergy (PDF format)
✐ *www.rci.rutgers.edu/~donas/ g-epi/Reading16.pdf*

Food Allergy Resources
✐ *www.efanet.org/activities/ documents/adversereactions tofood.pdf*

Information about Allergy Shots
✐ *www.aaaai.org/patients/pub- licedmat/tips/whatareallergy shots.stm*

Information on Pediatric Asthma

NIH Pediatric Asthma Compendium
✐ *www.nlm.nih.gov/medline plus/asthmainchildren.html*

Acne Care for Your Child

Acne Tips from the Department of Health and Human Services
✐ *www.niams.nih.gov/hi/ topics/acne/acne.htm*

Taking Care of Cuts and Bites

Over-the-Counter Wound-Care from the FDA
✐ *www.fda.gov/fdac/features/ 496_cuts.html*

Treating Spider Bites
✐ *www.calpoison.org/ public/spiders.html*

DEET Safety for Parents
✐ *www.aap.org/family/ wnv-jun03.htm*

Cold Remedies and Your Child

The Danger of Over-the-Counter Cough and Cold Medications
✐ *www.pediatrics.org/ cgi/content/full/108/3/e52*

Orthopedic Conditions in Children

Information on Scoliosis from the Mayo Clinic
✐ *www.mayoclinic.com/ health/scoliosis/DS00194*

Index

THE EVERYTHING®
PARENT'S GUIDES SERIES

Expert Advice for Parents in Need of Answers

All titles are trade paperback, 6" x 9", $14.95

The Everything® Parent's Guide to Raising a Successful Child
ISBN 10: 1-59337-043-1; ISBN 13: 978-1-59337-043-5

The Everything® Parent's Guide to Children with Autism
ISBN 10: 1-59337-041-5; ISBN 13: 978-1-59337-041-1

The Everything® Parent's Guide to Children with Bipolar Disorder
ISBN 10: 1-59337-446-1; ISBN 13: 978-1-59337-446-4

The Everything® Parent's Guide to Children with Dyslexia
ISBN 10: 1-59337-135-7; ISBN 13: 978-1-59337-135-7

The Everything® Parent's Guide to Children with
Asperger's Syndrome
ISBN 10: 1-59337-153-5; ISBN 13: 978-1-59337-153-1

The Everything® Parent's Guide to Tantrums
ISBN 10: 1-59337-321-X; ISBN 13: 978-1-59337-321-4

The Everything® Parent's Guide to Children with ADD/ADHD
ISBN 10: 1-59337-308-2; 978-1-59337-308-5

The Everything® Parent's Guide to Positive Discipline
ISBN 10: 1-58062-978-4; ISBN 13: 978-1-58062-978-2

THE EVERYTHING® PARENT'S GUIDES SERIES (CONTINUED).

The Everything® Parent's Guide to the Strong-Willed Child
ISBN 10: 1-59337-381-3; ISBN 13: 978-1-59337-381-8

The Everything® Parent's Guide to Raising Siblings
ISBN 10: 1-59337-537-9; ISBN 13: 978-1-59337-537-9

The Everything® Parent's Guide to Sensory Integration Disorder
ISBN 10: 1-59337-714-2; ISBN 13: 978-1-59337-714-4

The Everything® Parent's Guide to Children and Divorce
ISBN 10: 1-59337-418-6; ISBN 13: 978-1-59337-418-1

The Everything® Parent's Guide to Raising Boys
ISBN 10: 1-59337-587-5; ISBN 13: 978-1-59337-587-4

The Everything® Parent's Guide to Childhood Illnesses
ISBN 10: 1-59869-239-9; ISBN 13: 978-1-59869-239-6

The Everything® Parent's Guide to Raising Girls
ISBN 10: 1-59869-247-X; ISBN 13: 978-1-59869-247-1

The Everything® Parent's Guide to Children with Juvenile Diabetes
ISBN 10: 1-59869-246-1; ISBN 13: 978-1-59869-246-4

The Everything® Parent's Guide to Children with Depression
ISBN 10: 1-59869-264-X; ISBN 13: 978-1-59869-264-8

Everything® and Everything.com® are registered trademarks of
F&W Publications, Inc.